The Barns Experiment

Originally published in 1945, this is a concise account of the remarkable experiment with boys carried out by the author of *The Hawkspur Experiment*. The war put this latter experiment into abeyance, but gave its author an opportunity to practice his principles on a group of younger difficult boys. Aged from eight to fourteen, these boys were the "throw-outs" of the Evacuation Scheme, but before the Barns experiment had been long in operation troublesome boys were being evacuated not primarily to escape bombs, but in order that they might have the treatment that Barns provided.

Barns was a Hostel-school initiated by the Society of Friends, where lawless boys made their own laws, and where the principle instrument in their reformation was not punishment but affection. So successful were the unconventional methods here described that sceptics were convinced, and Barns has now achieved a permanent place in the field of "the therapy of the dis-social." Today it would be described as a therapeutic community and is one of the earliest experiments of its kind that raised awareness and paved the way for further research in this area.

The Barns Experiment

W. David Wills

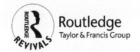

Routledge
Taylor & Francis Group

First published in 1945
by George Allen and Unwin Ltd

This edition first published in 2023 by Routledge
4 Park Square, Milton Park, Abingdon, Oxon, OX14 4RN

and by Routledge
605 Third Avenue, New York, NY 10017

Routledge is an imprint of the Taylor & Francis Group, an informa business

© 1945 W. David Wills

Publisher's Note
The publisher has gone to great lengths to ensure the quality of this reprint but points out that some imperfections in the original copies may be apparent.

Disclaimer
The publisher has made every effort to trace copyright holders and welcomes correspondence from those they have been unable to contact.

A Library of Congress record exists under LCCN: 46002425

ISBN: 978-1-032-41046-3 (hbk)
ISBN: 978-1-003-35602-8 (ebk)
ISBN: 978-1-032-41058-6 (pbk)

Book DOI 10.4324/9781003356028

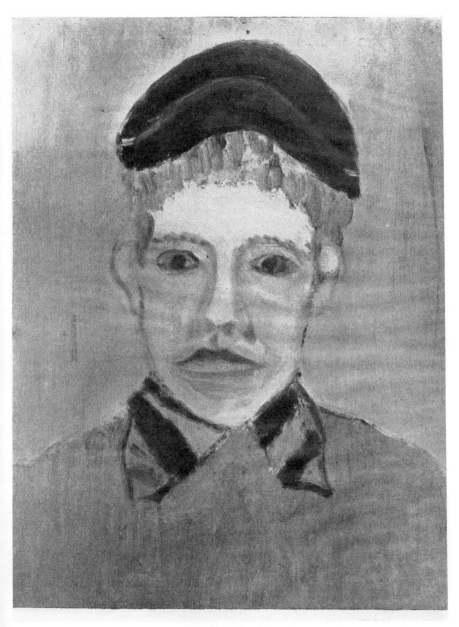

SAMMIE JOHNSON
Self portrait

THE
BARNS EXPERIMENT

by

W. DAVID WILLS

My Course, by the will of God, has

had something of a method in it,

which makes the telling more easy

JOHN BUCHAN *John Burnet of Barns*

London

GEORGE ALLEN AND UNWIN LTD

Museum Street

FIRST PUBLISHED IN 1945
SECOND IMPRESSION 1947

PRINTED IN GREAT BRITAIN
in 11-point Baskerville, leaded
BY C. TINLING & CO., LTD.
LIVERPOOL, LONDON, AND PRESCOT

PREFACE

I HAVE tried to write a book that he who runs may read. I have, therefore, tried to avoid the use of words that might send the general reader running to his dictionary, only to find that they are not there because they are not English, but the esoteric jargon of the psychologist. I hope that any such of the cognoscenti as may read it will forgive what may seem to them an over simplification of concepts that cannot easily be expressed in everyday English.

Everyday English it is indeed, for it has had to be a book that he who runs has *written*. Hastily scribbled in snatched half-hours and brief holidays, it has no more claim to elegance of style than to erudition of matter. In this, too, I hope I may be indulged.

For it is a tale, I feel, that needs to be told. One of its earliest critics, who read part of the manuscript, asked : "Who is it intended for ? " and perhaps this is the place to answer that question. It is intended to "Strengthen such as do stand ; and to comfort and help the weak-hearted." The kind of approach to problems of juvenile behaviour which I have here outlined is one that, while still in its infancy, is become a fairly lusty infant. But there are those who (whether using, or merely interested in this approach) are oppressed by the difficulties, both of application and opposition, and I hope they may derive some help and encouragement from the perusal of our experience at Barns.

But that is not all. In a democratic society such as ours aspires to be, nothing is entirely the province of the specialist, and true progress is a plant whose roots reach wide and deep among an informed and enlightened populace. I want indeed to see the arm of those who attempt to use this kind of method strengthened, but that is best done by the sustenance of public approval. The public can approve only what it knows ; this book is an attempt to help in the dissemination of that necessary knowledge.

I shall have frequent recurrence in what follows to the first person singular. There are two reasons for this. One is simply that I find that mode of writing easiest. The other is that I have given frequent expression to opinions for which I have not sought the concurrence of my colleagues. Our work has involved the co-operation of a number of different bodies including Public Authorities, such as the Peeblesshire County Council, who are quite innocent of any measure of responsibility for the method

employed, and whom I should not like to saddle with the guilt of
heterodoxy, whether of action or of opinion. This is not, let me
hasten to add, to diminish in any way the invaluable support I have
received from a wide variety of bodies and persons ; and the less
they were committed to the principles on which I have been working,
the greater the credit that is due to them for the help and encouragement they have given. To attempt to thank them all—The Society
of Friends ; members and officials of the Peeblesshire County
Council and the Edinburgh Corporation ; the officials of the
Departments of Health and Education for Scotland ; the W.V.S. ;
the Barns House Committee of Management and my immediate
colleagues at Barns ; as well as the host of people who have sustained
our work in a private capacity ; would make a list as tedious as a
shorter list would be invidious.

To two persons, however, I must make particular reference.
To thank them would be presumptuous, for their concern for the
ends we have sought and their interest in their achievement is no
less than mine. But to our Chairman, Mary F. Smith (Mrs. Lionel
Smith), I will not be denied the satisfaction of attempting to express
something of my feelings of gratitude, respect and affection which
each of the four years of our collaboration has increased. Nor can
I be prevented from speaking in the same terms of my wife, whose
unwavering support has enhanced those feelings not during four,
but fourteen years of faithful comradeship.

CONTENTS

ILLUSTRATIONS

The following pages will be found to contain many hard sayings about mothers. If my standard seems impossibly high, I must lay the blame on her to whom I dedicate this book

SUSAN EMILY WILLS

a very pattern among mothers.

CHAPTER ONE

EARLY DAYS

" And certainly there *was* a most extraordinary noise going on within—a constant howling and sneezing, and every now and then a great crash, as if a dish or kettle had been broken to pieces."

LEWIS CARROLL—" Alice's Adventures in Wonderland."

DINNER is finished, and the President rings the bell for silence. He is thirteen years old, and makes a very good President, though inclined to be a little self-righteous.

" Any announcements ? " Several hands go up, including that of Ben Stoddard, the head teacher. He wishes to say that after school is over to-day, there will be extra school for any who want it. There is general approbation of this, and a shout of " Hurray " from Johnnie Bellger.

Sammy has something to say—" I'm charging Ben Stoddard for bullying me in school this morning." Ruth wants to say there will be painting at three o'clock for as many as will, and one of the orderly squad wants to say—" Will you please pass your plates to the end of the table." Then the President touches his bell again, and there is a stampede for the door.

The casual visitor may think it a very strange establishment where a boy of thirteen controls a dining room of thirty boys and seven or eight adults ; where a boy cheers at the prospect of extra school ; and where a child of ten can bring a " charge " of bullying against his teacher without exciting comment. Indeed, there is much that is unusual about this community of thirty " difficult" boys and their attendant adults, though it has all become commonplace to us who live there.

That charge of bullying, for instance—it might be interesting to the uninitiated to follow it up.

Although all charges must be announced at dinner time, they are not heard until a few hours later, at the Committee, sitting round a table in the Dining Room. Here, the Minister of Justice presides (age 11) and it is rather an imposing body as it consists of all the ministers. An adult has been asked on this occasion to attend and record the findings because, the Minister of Justice says, " My writing's not so good."

" Go on then, Sammy ! "

" I'm charging Ben for shaking me in school this morning."

9

"What happened?"

"Well, he said I was'na getting on with ma work, an' I said I was, and he shook me—he shook me hard; made me greet." (It is to be observed that he is far from greeting now; seems in fact to be thoroughly enjoying himself).

"Have you anything to say, Ben?"

"Well, I'm afraid its true I shook Sammy."

"*Why* did you shake him?"

"I'm afraid it's a long story, and it goes back a long way. Do you want to hear it all?"

"Aye, we'll hear it."

"All right. We all know that Sammy has a lot of trouble over his school work, especially his reading. It is not his fault—he missed school over a year through being in hospital—but there you are, he *is* behind. Well, there's nothing remarkable about that. Several boys are behind without having been in hospital. They know they're behind, but it doesn't worry them. They want to catch up, so when we have extra school in the afternoon they come along. But Sammy somehow can't bear to admit that he's behind. He thinks it's something to be ashamed of. Then he's so afraid of finding something he can't do in the work that's set him that he refuses to do it, and says I've set something he can't be *expected* to do, before he's even looked at it. This is nothing new—it's been going on a long time now, and it's been the cause of no end of trouble in the class-room, because Sammy isn't content with saying he can't do things—he has to show there are things he *can* do by making himself a nuisance to everyone. I haven't complained to the Committee or the Minister of School because I realise it's something the Committee can't deal with very well—it's something we must just hope Sammy will get out of by degrees, like other boys have. But it *has* caused a lot of trouble, and this morning it caused even more than usual. Instead of getting on with his work, Sammy was just pestering everyone, and those who were anxious to get on with the job found it almost impossible. At last I shifted his desk away from the others, but he refused to stay there, and made himself such an insufferable nuisance that at last I lost patience with him and —well, I shook him. It wasn't a good thing to do, and I'm afraid I was rather hasty. But I can't deny that I shook him." A painful silence ensues. All feel—indeed, all *know*—that Ben endured considerable provocation. They realise too, that if the matter of Sammy's misbehaviour had been brought before them by the Minister of School there was precious little they could have done about it. You can't *compel* a boy to enjoy school like the others.

But then—we can't have shakings. As the Minister of Money says, *sotto voce*, to the Minister of Justice, there's been a lot of bullying by the Staff lately. So Ben is ordered to pay Sammy sixpence "damages"—and the next case comes on.

I have told this story because I hope it might reproduce something of the atmosphere of Barns. Not that charges of bullying by the staff are common occurrences ; they are a rarity because we are opposed to the use of any kind of violence. And it must not be thought that this atmosphere existed from the start. It had to be created in the face of a good deal of opposition—much of it from the boys themselves ! I was asked once by a critic (one, who, incidentally, later became much less critical) whether the boys liked our methods, or whether they preferred the more orthodox kind of discipline that they were used to. I had to reply that they probably preferred the more orthodox kind of discipline (at any rate at first) and went on to use the well known disciplinarian argument that what they *like* is not necessarily what is good for them.

They were all difficult boys, hating school, prejudiced against adults in general, punished often but not wisely, fearful, suspicious, aggressive, untruthful, uncared for and, in the main, unloved. During the early days of Barns they were their own worst enemies because they strove hard to compel us to furnish them with the only kind of security they knew—the security of outward compulsion ; and we were determined to give them security on a different level —the security that comes from the knowledge of being loved.

We refused to use any kind of punishment, and as soon as the boys began to suspect that this was our intention, they naturally began to put it to the test. At the beginning of the Autumn Term, 1940, there were six boys ; by the end of the term there were about thirty. Each new accretion of boys (they generally came in groups of four or five) set out to find "punishment point" and the chaos and disorder can perhaps be imagined. Or perhaps not. The atmosphere in those days was one of surging unrest. The chief game seemed to consist of charging wildly through the house howling madly and slamming all the doors on the way. Any kind of organised activity was almost impossible. Crockery would be dashed on to stone floors, games destroyed, furniture broken, stones hurled through windows. Mealtimes were an indescribable babel, and there were mass truantings from school.

They had never before met people whose instructions were not accompanied by threats, open or implied, and they were upset by it. We cannot blame them. Threats of punishment are so woven into the weft of our daily life that we take them for granted, and hardly notice that they are there. I wonder how many laws there are on the Statute Book—or by-laws in the local annals—that do not contain a threat ? From the laws forbidding me to kill English-men and requiring me to kill Germans, to the by-laws saying, "One way only" or "Do not Spit ; penalty forty shillings." And I wonder what the reaction of the ordinary decent citizen would be if he awoke one morning to find all these sanctions gone ? I do wonder very much indeed.

I think Jean Penman, our first House Matron, probably had the worst of it. She could tell some tales that are—in retrospect—very amusing. She had charge of a group of the youngest boys, who slept together in one dormitory. One little imp (it was Ian Burns, I think) tried every conceivable kind of wickedness to provoke Jean to punish him, ending at last one night by getting quietly into bed saying, "This is a funny place. You *never* get the belt ! " Not that that was the end of his troubles, by any means. He found after a while that he could get the belt at school—but that is another story. It was about this boy, too, I believe, that Jean came to me for advice once, because his tantrums and violence and general unpleasantness would soon, she feared, be "getting her down." I gave her, so far as I remember, two alternative lots of advice. One was a counsel of perfection—to remain unmoved and unangered, and to be consistently affectionate. This being, as I thought, impossible, I went on to make some less idealistic, but more practicable suggestions ; I forget now what they were. But Jean chose the hard way (that is the kind of colleague I have had) and was delighted with the results shewn in a few weeks' time. Then there was a boy whose chief delight was to pounce on the back of some unsuspecting female and hammer her with all his strength. Jean asked him if he did that to everyone. " No," he said, "Only to those I like." And he spoke the truth. The door of Jean's room still bears the scars of those days.

The astonishing thing was that it all ended quite suddenly. At the end of the first term they were as wild and unruly and unresponsive as ever ; by the beginning of the second they seemed like different boys. I say "seemed" because I doubt whether the casual visitor would have been very much impressed by their outward behaviour even then. But we who lived with them knew that something had happened. They were convinced of our sincerity, and were ready to accept us. They were still the same boys, still needing a tremendous amount of love and skilled attention before they could return to the outside world without fear of danger to themselves or their neighbours—but the cure could now begin ; they were no longer in opposition.

This stage had not taken as long as I expected. I had reckoned on a minimum of six months, and it took four. But no sooner had the opposition of the boys been overcome than we found ourselves faced with a different and more formidable opposition. To tell of this I must explain something of the administrative " set-up " by which Barns was conducted.

The Public Authority immediately responsible for Barns as an Evacuation Hostel was the Peeblesshire County Council, which, however, worked through a Committee of Management consisting mainly of members of the Society of Friends (which had initiated the scheme), and on this Committee the County Council was represented by its Chairman. It is to this Committee that I have been responsible, and a happier relationship could hardly exist. Technically, I am their employee, doing a piece of work on their behalf ; in practice our relationship, perhaps to the outsider a curious one, but common enough in the Society of Friends is that of a Committee " liberating " a man to do a piece of work for which he is " under concern." Their support and encouragement have been constant and unfailing.

This Committee of Management appointed me, and it also appointed such of the staff as are paid by the County Council. These are a House matron, a sub-warden, a cook-housekeeper and domestic workers who have varied in number from time to time. In the interests of efficiency there has been a necessary degree of division of labour, but there has never been any kind of social distinction between the various types of worker. To say that we have lived together as a family is trite but truthful.

In so far, however, as all boys came from Edinburgh, and the Edinburgh Education Authority paid the teaching staff, that body also had an interest in Barns but was not (I do not know why ; it just wasn't thought of at the time) was not represented on the Committee and was therefore not so familiar with what was going on. That is not to say that they were in any sense antipathetic, but merely that they, and the teacher they seconded to us, maintained an attitude of friendly reserve until we should have proved ourselves. He—the teacher—was a scientist, and confessed to an attitude of scientific detachment. He would be interested, he said, to see how it worked. But in a venture of faith such as ours was, scientific detachment was not enough. It was all very well for the bystander to take that attitude, but among those actually engaged in the work, who is not for us, is against us. When, therefore, at the end of the first term he went to his employers and complained of the difficulties of his job, not the least of which was trying to maintain order in school when such " license " was permitted outside it, I was not in the least surprised. Indeed, I had written to the Authority immediately on his appointment and had told them to expect this very thing.

Nor could anyone blame him for being somewhat dissatisfied. He had to teach, single-handed, thirty boys of widely varying ages and capacities, all of whom were there because they were " difficult." We had no domestic workers at that time so the help that we were able to offer him would have been very little, even if he had felt more able to make use of it than he did.

But this well justified and reluctant opposition from within the camp was not all. Other and more disturbing reports had reached the Education Authority at about the same time. Official visitors had been to Barns from the Juvenile Court, and had submitted a " condemnatory " report in which they had expressed the view that they did not consider Barns a place to which they could refer their cases. That did not worry us, because we did not want Court cases. But the opinion of these visitors could hardly· be ignored by the Education Authority.

Here was opposition indeed, and if some members of the Education Committee were inclined to attribute all our alleged failings to our obstinate refusal to punish wrongdoers, I do not think we can very well blame them. " A strap behind the door, Mr. Wills," said one of them—not without a certain amount of heat—" you should keep a strap behind the door." Their teacher took their advice—indeed, he had specifically asked to be excused from using our methods, and from that time corporal punishment was a regular feature of his department of our work, and remained so until Ben Stoddard took charge of the school at the end of 1942.

But the Edinburgh Education Authority, while properly supporting their employee, were not prepared to condemn us merely on the word of the visiting dignitaries to whom I have referred. There was a conference in which we were given an opportunity to explain what we were up to and, while they were unable to accept our point of view, they were not prepared to condemn it. Some weeks later there was a visit by the whole of the Committee responsible for primary schools in Edinburgh. If we did not succeed in removing the last lingering doubt of every member of that Committee, at least we removed all doubts in the mind of the Chairman of the Education Committee, who wrote me a charming letter immediately on his return in order to tell me so. When, therefore, at the end of the first year the question of appointing a half-time teacher arose they were quite prepared to accept our nominee, Ben Stoddard, and raised no objection when, a year later, we recommended that he replace the teacher-in-charge who was returning to Edinburgh.

I could say much more, and some of it very amusing about the opposition we experienced in our early days, but there is very little point in doing so. The reason for referring to it at all is simply this : One of my objects in writing this account of our work is that perhaps others may be stimulated or encouraged to go and do likewise. If they do, they must realise that they, too, will almost certainly have the same sort of opposition to overcome in their early days, especially if they allow it to be known that they do not punish. There are many people—and they are to be found in all walks of society—whose worst passions seem to be aroused by the idea of a boy not being spanked and of a school being run without a strap. These people are not merely contemptuous—which one could understand—they are sometimes even venomous. And even among the less venomous ; even, indeed, among the friendliest of critics ; there is an extraordinary proneness to assume that there are only two alternatives—*either* a child is punished, *or* he is allowed to do exactly as he likes. To them it seems inconceivable that a child can be unpunished and yet not be licentious. They seem never to have heard of a force which rules its kingdom without a sword !

Perhaps I should deal now with this thorny question of punishment and get it out of the way ; but there is one simple recipe for overcoming all the opposition that will be met in carrying on such work as ours. You simply need an unflinching faith in the methods you are using and a certain measure of patience. Without them you had better not start.

CHAPTER TWO

PUNISHMENT

" . . . at this day it is still resorted to by cunning and malignant savages in Australia, Africa and *Scotland*." *
SIR JAMES FRAZER—" The Golden Bough."

" WHERE the deuce are you getting all that wood from ? " I said one day to a gang of boys who were stacking a pile of beautiful logs outside the back door. " From the playing-field," they said. Actually they meant from a piece of land adjacent to the playing-field, where a wood had been felled a couple of years previously. " I don't think we'd better use that," I said, " It doesn't belong to us." " Shall we get into a row then ? " " No, as a matter of fact, I don't think there's any danger of a *row*. I don't suppose for a moment that the Estate want this wood—it's only scrap timber, and it's quite on the cards they'll be glad to have it cleared away. But we don't *know* that, and anyway, the point is that it's not ours, and we've no right to take it away without permission." And congratulating myself on my calm and reasonable attitude, I went about my business. An hour later I was astonished to find an even larger gang of boys, still carrying logs from the " playing-field." " What the heck *is* this," I said, " I thought I told you to leave that wood alone." " You didna. You said it was all right to take it." " *I* said it was all right ? You're dreaming "—" You said we shouldn't get a row."

This kind of thing leaves me speechless, and it is going on all the time. The moral question is one that does not seem to exist for our boys. They do not disregard it—they are merely unaware of it. So far as Right and Wrong mean anything at all to the boys at Barns they seem only to mean " not punishable " and " punishable." I heard one little boy talking in a self-righteous way about not being a thief, and I asked him why not. He replied indignantly that *he* didn't want to go to an Approved School. " But surely," I said, " a smart boy like you could do a little nicking without being found out ? " But no, he didn't seem to feel that one could ever be safe from detection. I pressed him further, and asked other boys who were near why they shouldn't steal. Never once

---

* The italics are mine ; and it is only fair to say that the eminent Scot was not referring to the same barbarous practice as that about which I am writing.

did anything approaching a moral reason rear its head. Or perhaps once, when one boy, seeing that I was looking for a specific answer tried, " It might get Barns a bad name," to see if that was what I wanted him to say. Even him I had to discourage by pointing out that it would only " get Barns a bad name " if it were found out. It occurred to no one to say simply that it was wrong to steal, or that it isn't fair, or it's not very nice for the person from whom the theft is made. The only question to be considered before taking any course of action is " Will anyone do anything to me," and if the answer to that question is in the affirmative, then there is the supplementary question—" Shall I be found out ? " Our aim at Barns is to provide a somewhat higher motive for conduct.

" I had sooner have a plain russet-coated Captain," said Oliver Cromwell, " That knows what he fights for and loves what he knows, than that which you call a gentleman and is nothing else." This is a dictum with a wider relevance than Cromwell gave it. The finest type of citizen is he who obeys no law blindly out of an unthinking respect for authority or fear of penalties ; it is he whose conduct is based on a rational understanding of why a given type of behaviour is desirable, and who will persist in that type of behaviour whatever the consequences to himself. Such a citizen will not always be strictly " law-abiding," because he will be prepared if necessary to defy a law which he considers unjust or harmful to the best interests of Society. No State or Community can hope to achieve or continue in true greatness when it ceases to breed such citizens. And such citizens cannot be bred in a Society which uses fear as its chief instrument in the training of the young.

This is the basis of my opposition to the use of punishment in general, as distinct from those reasons which have a particular relevance to the treatment of delinquency. It is not the fundamental reason for my non-penal attitude—the fundamental reason is that I consider punishment contrary to Christian teaching, whatever its expediency ; but as even Christians do not agree on this point, I shall concern myself for the moment with empirical, rather than religious or moral reasons. About the latter, I hope to write later ; in the meantime I return to those reasons which it seems to me should be acceptable to the intelligent man, whatever his religious beliefs.

If I were to base my own conduct in eschewing punishment at the lowest level, I should say that it has been tried on the boys with whom I am concerned, and it has not worked. Strictly speaking, of course, it has not been tried at all, as I understand it. Perhaps if the boys had been punished efficiently they might not have come to us. But they have—for the most part—merely been smacked or

B

knocked about for doing things that caused annoyance or inconvenience to their elders.

I was occasionally punished myself, as a child ; sometimes even spanked. And, like the Blimps who favour birching because they were flogged at Eton or Harrow, I don't know that I am any the worse for it. But my father is a deeply religious man with a very strong moral sense ; perhaps too strong, though I become increasingly doubtful about that as I get older. When he felt it his duty to spank ; for that matter, when he simply lost his temper ; it was quite clear to me that the spanking was a sign of his deep horror of something I had done. It is not facetious to say that words (that I could understand) were not adequate to express his feelings about what I had done, though I am prepared to concede that exasperation may have been a contributory cause of his difficulties of articulation. He felt himself compelled to have recourse to a procedure that I *could* understand. Although I often re-acted violently on these occasions, and called my father many hard names, I do not think I was ever conscious for long of any personal animus. I always realised that the horror and the spanking were directed against the swearing or whatever, and not against me. It was a process of conditioning. That particular offence was associated in my mind with an unpleasant experience and I came therefore to regard the offence as an unpleasant thing. To this day, though I sometimes swear mildly myself, and though I have lived most of my life in company where there was a good deal of swearing ; though I can see no rational objection to bad language except on æsthetic grounds ; even now, I cannot overcome the horror of certain words that was thus bred in me. Perhaps it was overdone, but at any rate it was done, and in that sense was infinitely more justifiable than the casual and irrational beatings to which many of our boys have been subjected. I have no wish to defend this method of moral education, however many excellent men it may have produced in the past ; but if we are to abandon the method of conditioning by fear we must make sure we have got something to put in its place. In so many homes parents try to be "progressive" and, avoiding the use of punishment, assume that they must allow their children to do just whatever they like at all times. Their friends and relations, seeing the children growing up into nastly little savages say, " These progressive methods, my dear ! " and we who try to find a better weapon than fear are collectively damned.

But these Barns boys are not in the " never been smacked" class. They have been smacked well and often, but the smacking has

not been " tied up " with the offence—there has been no conditioning—except against the parents and all adults. So far as
there has been any smacking or other punishment for acts that were
wrong, and not merely a source of annoyance, they have often been
accompanied by a snigger of pride at the child's " devilishness "—
not a bad thing in itself, but of course no trouble is ever taken to let
the child understand what it all means. What is the result of all this?
I have told you how Ian Burns said, "This is a funny place—you
never get the belt." The same boy was standing by when I was telling
a group of boys that some people thought I ought to use a belt on
them. "Why do they say that?" asked Ian, " Don't they like us?"

Whatever may be the effect of punishment on other children,
there is no doubt that to children coming from the sort of homes from
which most of the Barns boys come, a person who deliberately
hurts you cannot be a person who loves you. As love is fundamental to our therapy, we must obviously avoid anything which
might give a contrary impression. So we cannot use punishment.

We had during one period at Barns a long series of " unsolved
crimes." They consisted for the most part of thefts of money from
adults. Many of the threads that were taken up in trying to solve
them seemed to lead to Stephen Baillie, and his behaviour became
more and more suspicious. He started talking to people about
his " hidy-holes," and saying where he would hide ten shillings if he
had it, and so forth. Eventually, he was taxed with having done
some of the stealing. His reply was, " What if I have ? " I asked
him what he meant by that. " Well—what can you do to me if I
have stolen it ? " I told him I wasn't concerned with doing things
to him—I only wanted to get the money back for the people to whom
it belonged, and who couldn't afford to lose it. He then denied
very firmly all knowledge of the matter, and as I had nothing
" against him " but his own half-incriminating suggestions, I had to
let it drop. Presently, however, fresh evidence came to light.
Some boys claimed that Stephen had told them that he had some
money hidden in one of his " hidy-holes " down by the river. I
questioned them carefully and there seemed no doubt that he had
said this, though none of them had actually seen the money. I got
hold of Stevie again and asked him if he had said this. He made
no attempt to deny it. " Is it the stolen money ? " No reply.
" It *is* the stolen money then ? " . . . " Well—what if it is ? "
" If it is, you'd better go and get it, pronto." After some hesitation
and humming and hawing, he went. Half-an-hour passed, and I
went to see how he was getting on. He claimed to be unable to
find the hole. I helped him (with a very bad grace) to search,

and it soon became clear that there was no hole anywhere near where we were searching. Then he said that perhaps it wasn't there but somewhere else, and in short led me on a very long wild goose chase, to the great detriment of that judicial calm which I so often advocate, but so rarely achieve. Eventually, exasperated and fuming, I gave it up, in a state of profound sympathy with that type of person who is most likely to disagree with the contentions of this chapter.

Stevie had never taken any of the money at all, and half our difficulties in finding the culprit had been due to his efforts to direct suspicion to himself. Stevie was, it is true, doing his fair share of stealing about this time, but being unable to secure enough (or indeed any) punishment by his own petty pilfering, he tried to take the blame for this more serious stealing, because *he wanted to be punished*. Is there anything to be gained by punishing such a boy as this?—even when he *is* guilty? You may think Stevie's an outstanding case, but as one can never be sure how far this element enters into a boy's behaviour, it is obviously best to avoid punishment altogether.

The curious attitude of the punishment-seeker arises, from a deep-seated feeling of guilt, due very often to having " wicked" feelings about one's parents. Most of us have an ambivalent attitude to our parents—we hate them as well as love them— but while most of us by repression or otherwise dispose of the hatred without much difficulty, it may, where it is very strong, give rise to strong feelings of guilt and a desire to be punished for our wicked feelings. Stevie's case was a more than usually interesting one, for he had " killed " his father in fantasy. Obviously the way to deal with this situation is not to keep on assuaging the guilt-feeling by continual doses of punishment, but to eliminate the guilt feeling.

Stevie's may be an interesting, but it is not an exceptional case. Consider the story of Jacob Everson, who has to be numbered among our failures. When Jacob first came he seemed a sweet rosy-cheeked wee thing, though not always strictly truthful. After a few days he started running away home. He always returned in a day or two quite happily, and it was always difficult to find any reason why he ran away. When asked he would say, " I wanted to see if my mother was all right "—" Why shouldn't she be all right ? " I would ask, to which he would reply that there might have been an air-raid (I may add that he hardly ever went home without being infected with scabies). Over-solicitude of this kind is a sure sign of ambivalence—trying to make up for the hate by giving evidence of love. It may even, indeed, be that he had " killed " his mother in an imaginary air-raid, and he wanted to re-assure himself that she was not really dead. However, that may be, the ambivalence was duly noted. As we make a point of never appearing shocked when boys say unorthodox things about their parents, it was not very long before Jacob was telling someone quite casually, in the course of conversation, that he hated his " old woman," and in one way or another the fact of the ambivalence was firmly established.

It was one thing to recognise the ambivalence ; quite another to deal with it effectively, especially when it appeared that he hated both his parents intensely. This was a case for psychotherapy, but war circumstances made that impossible. I did the little bit of psychological first-aid that I allow myself to do in such circumstances. I encouraged him to talk about his parents and so far from appearing shocked when he sometimes said unpleasant things about them, I let him know that this was not such a frightfully uncommon or shocking thing, that other people had such feelings, that it didn't mean he didn't love them, and so forth. The effect of these surface proddings is doubtful, but at any rate so long as one doesn't start talking a lot of psychological clap-trap (such a temptation to the amateur psychologist !) it does no harm, and one feels that no stone should be unturned.

In such a case it seems to me that the first essential is that the desire to be punished should not be met (except, perhaps, sometimes in a token way) so that the psyche is compelled to seek some other resolution of the conflict (the conflict, *i.e.*, between the hate felt for the parent and the desire to be " good "). In such circumstances any suggestion falls upon open ears and an open mind, and one may even hope that " environmental" treatment of the right kind will in time alone bring about the required adjustment. But if the guilt feeling is being periodically appeased by doses of punishment, a rough and ready adjustment has been made, and it is immeasurably more difficult to interest the person concerned in finding another. It is here that we laboured under a difficulty with Jacob. When he began to be naughty, we refused to punish him. His delinquencies increased, but we were not to be moved. Then he discovered the weak chink in our armour. The Head teacher could be persuaded to oblige—and did oblige. This solved the problem for a time ; he became a very well-conducted boy in the House because he was just being naughty enough in school to get an occasional punishment. Then Ben came along and wrecked everything. He was Assistant teacher at first, and Jacob was put into his class—where, of course, there was no punishment. It was about this time that he became Chairman of the Citizens' Association, and an outstanding member of the Community. But though he was such an outstanding success in the House he was a great nuisance to Ben as he still expected to get his dose of medicine at school, where he now sometimes behaved himself so badly as to fetch in the Head from the next room. But he couldn't get enough that way, and anyway, the summer holidays—seven weeks of them—came along with no hope of punishment. It was then that he committed an " extra-mural " crime. I will not go into details of how I became an accessory after the fact, in order to hide this crime (though taking care to see that no one was the loser by it) and of how èven then he concealed part of his offence in the hope that the Police would get track of it. But we managed to foil all that, and took jolly good care to see that he didn't get another opportunity for an " outside job "—if I may reverse the usual meaning of that phrase. Then followed, during the autumn, a really determined attempt either to secure punishment or to get sent away from Barns so that he would be able to get it somewhere else. There was a long series of really serious offences—stealing largish sums from staff-rooms by means of most daring and clever expedients—tinkering with locks, using fire escapes and what not. During one period there was hardly a night that he was not abroad in the house. It was a difficult and a critical period, but a hopeful one. But he beat us in the end. While Head teacher was away at Christmas, Jacob (with another boy in very similar case) burgled his cottage and went off with a number of valuables, and all the Head's belts. They carefully left behind them a little toy tank which everyone knew belonged to one of them, as if to destroy any lingering element of doubt, and the Head—as they had guessed—thought it his duty to inform the Police. Foolishly, as I now see, I advised the. parents to keep the boys at home in the hope of mitigating the severity of the Court. But they have both subsequently reached their desired haven, and are both now in Approved Schools, in spite of the patience—the too much patience—of the Courts.

If a boy is committing a crime in order to be punished, how will he be stopped by punishing him ?

We have thus, so far, four reasons, each of which seems to me a perfectly sound reason why punishment should be avoided :—

   1. It establishes a base motive for conduct.

   2. It has been tried, and has failed ; or alternatively, it has been so mis-used in the past as to destroy its usefulness now.

3. It militates against the establishment of the relationship which we consider necessary between staff and children—a relationship in which the child must feel himself to be loved.

4. Many delinquent children (and adults) are seeking punishment as a means of assuaging their guilt-feelings.

But that is not all ; there is still another. When the offender has " paid for " his crime, he can " buy " another with an easy conscience. Who has not met the person who, on being found out, says, in an off-hand way, as if that closed the matter—" All right ! I'll take my punishment "—as if the expiation of the crime had entirely wiped it out ; as if by hanging the murderer, his victims were automatically returned to the bosom of his family. No one thinks that of course, but many are apt to act as if it were so. They talk about " taking the consequences of the crime." Only very rarely can a criminal do that—his victims have done it already. All the criminal can do is to take the consequences of being found out—a very different matter, which still leaves the victim bearing the consequences of the crime. It is like book-keeping. A crime is an entry on the credit side. When the punishment has been entered on the debit side the book is balanced and we are ready for the next credit entry. " What you people are trying to do," said someone, disparagingly, to a friend of mine, " is to take the risk out of wrong-doing ! " Exactly. A man may take a certain pride in doing a mean act for which he will have to endure punishment—" I can take it ! " If he cannot feel pride, he can justify it to his conscience by telling himself that, after all, he is prepared to take the consequences if the other side are smart enough to catch him. If you remove punishment you remove both the glamour and the false justification.

I may add, in parentheses, that this is one of the weaknesses of restitution. Sometimes when one of our boys has been hauled before the Committee for theft, he will try to pass it off grandly by saying airily, " I'll pay for it." That never satisfies me, and if I happen to be sitting in on the case (which is not very often) I always say, " What impertinence ! You pinch a bottle of ginger wine out of the stores, then you say to May (the cook), ' here's a tanner—go and buy yourself another.' Why should *she* have the fag of traipsing down to Peebles and hunting up a bottle of ginger wine and bringing it back here? I think he ought to replace a bottle of ginger wine, not just shell out some money."

But punishment is used in many schools and institutions for another reason than the " correction " of delinquency in the strict sense. It is used for the maintenance of discipline, and it seems to me that this is less easy to justify morally, but more easy to justify on grounds of expediency. By punishment inflicted to maintain discipline I mean, for example, giving a schoolboy the cane for impertinence. It is held that if the teacher is to carry out his duties effectively, he must be a rather distant person, set up on a pedestal of respect and authority, and commanding immediate obedience. He must be addressed as " Sir," and treated with respect. If a disrespectful attitude begins to shew itself it must immediately be stamped out, otherwise the foundations of the pedestals are undermined, and the teacher cannot effectively carry out his job.*

Now politeness and a respectful attitude to adults are very pleasing attributes—especially to the adults concerned. It is doubtful whether lack of them is so unmoral as to justify punishment, if punishment is ever justified. In such a case a child is made to suffer, not in order that he may become " good," but in order that authority may be maintained. This does not seem to me justifiable. We see the same practice in wider and more important spheres of human conduct. Soviet Russia, with great enlightenment, abolished the death penalty for ordinary crimes. But for crimes against the State—against discipline—thousands (if I may dare to say so of our fellow-fighter for freedom) have been executed merely on suspicion. Indeed, we do not need to go as far afield as Soviet Russia, as the position is much the same in our own country. Our severest penalties are reserved for murder and offences against the ultimate authority—" High Treason." Indeed, I can come closer home still, and give you the pleasure of having a dig at me. Last night the General Meeting at Barns House *outlawed* two boys who had defied the authority of the Vice-President (aged 13), on the grounds that the Vice-President had been speaking on behalf of the whole community. Outlawry is the severest penalty they have.

We at Barns (and by " we "—I mean now the adults) do not think we are entitled to make a child suffer in order to maintain our sacred prestige. It is difficult, if not impossible, to maintain this artificial prestige without making the children suffer, so we abandon it. I am Willsy (" Yer dinna say *sir* to 'im ! ") and the Head-teacher is Ben. Ben was explaining to some boys once that it was his duty to do something to which they were taking exception, because he was the teacher. " Garn," said one of them—" *You're*

---

* I believe it is commonly thought that this sort of thing is frightfully old-fashioned, and no longer done in any decent school. Don't you believe it. Writing, as I am, from Scotland, I may have a slightly prejudiced view of the matter. But I know precious few teachers in ordinary schools, either side of the border, who allow their pupils the same freedom of speech as they allow themselves.

no' a teacher ; you're just a man ! " Ben took this as a compliment, and I think he was right. Indeed, he said it was one of the best compliments he had had. It seems to me that this desire for artificial respect is an indication of pettiness and incompetence, as by its means " respect " may be—and often is—paid to the unrespectable. Whereas by our method only he (or she) is given respect who earns it—but it is real respect, and not a synthetic product compounded of fear and servility.

I said, though, that this reason for punishment is easy to defend on grounds of expediency. I was thinking of the poor elementary school teacher with forty to sixty children to teach all at once, often of very varying capacities. I confess that I cannot find it in my heart to blame a teacher who, in these circumstances, keeps " a strap behind the door." However dismally punishment may fail in making children " good," there is no doubt of its efficiency in keeping them quiet—though I have seen fools bungle that. I have heard of some teachers who, even in such circumstances, can keep order and do their job to all appearances successfully—without resort to punishment, but I confess that only one is known to me personally. Teaching, however, consists of more than keeping the class quiet, and it is doubtful how much real education takes place in a large class that is kept " in order " with the strap. I myself was one of a class of sixty, and while I should resist strenuously the charge of being completely uneducated, I owe precious little to my schooling, and I very much doubt whether the duller children ever learnt anything. Incidentally, when I was in the lower classes where the discipline was mild, I was always at the top of the class. When I moved up to a class where the discipline was severe, I slumped right down to the middle. There is not the slightest doubt in my mind that a class of more than thirty—at the very most—means that a number will not be taught, whatever the method. So while I consider punishment for the maintenance of discipline to be immoral, I can find it in my heart to forgive it in some circumstances. But I cannot condone the state of affairs which causes some excellent people to feel that they have no alternative.

What I cannot stand, however, is the widely-held belief that discipline so imposed is *good* for the children. To hold such a belief is merely to rationalise one's sadistic and self-aggrandising impulses. Discipline so maintained is a jolly good thing for the teacher—it makes life easier and more peaceful for him. It may have an incidental value to some of the children by enabling them to get on with their work. But I deny emphatically and absolutely that a child's character is enhanced by an imposed discipline. By an " imposed discipline," I mean the kind of " healthy discipline " one hears of in Approved Schools, Public Schools*, Boys' Brigades, Training Ships, and such institutions, where life (and not an unpleasant life necessarily, especially in retrospect) is ordered and arranged, every moment of the day mapped out and a rough and ready justice applied by the adults (or their quislings) for every departure from the established routine. My case against this kind of discipline is no different from anyone else's. First, it inhibits initiative. How can initiative develop in an atmosphere where all the initiating is done by the adults or others in authority, and all one is called upon to do is to conform ? Then it prevents the growth of self-reliance—one learns to rely on the system instead of on one's self, and by the same token it shifts responsibility for one's actions on to someone else. One never needs to enquire " Is this right or wrong," but only " Is this allowed ? " If it is not allowed, then it is someone else's duty to see that I don't do it—not *mine*. In short it thwarts, cramps and starves, and the only people who get any good out of it are those I have referred to (perhaps too severely) as the quislings of the system, who help the masters to impose their will as prefects, monitors, or what you will.

Here—and finally—to withhold you from hasty judgments, I must enter a caveat. However bad a thing " discipline " may be, a child does need to feel secure. He needs the loving care and solicitude of adults to advise, to teach, to warn and, if need be, to compel. It is an absolute law at Barns, laid down arbitrarily by me, and no humbug about it, that there is to be no bathing in the Tweed except in the presence of an adult. This law is upheld by the simple authority of my word, and attempts to break it are so rare as to be negligible. The presence of a strong adult who can lay down and maintain the law in this way is of inestimable benefit to a child in providing the necessary background of security. But that is all that is necessary—a background, not an all-pervading and inescapable atmosphere of rules, regulations, penalties and punishments. In front of this background there must be the maximum freedom for trial and error, struggle and achievement, work done or dodged, games played or wrecked, risks taken and dangers overcome. That is the sort of atmosphere that makes for sturdy growth, independence, initiative and manliness. That is the sort of atmosphere we strive after, at Barns.

* My knowledge of these institutions is based entirely on hearsay, but I am not disposed in their favour by what I have seen or heard of their products. Even Mr. Winston. Churchill who might to some seem an exception, was almost entirely self-educated while serving in the Army. (See " My Early Life," by Winston S. Churchill).

CHAPTER THREE

BARNS BOYS

" Shall I then drop the needle of insinuation and pick up the club of statement ? "
J. E. FLECKER-*Hassan*.

I HAVE spoken all this time in a vague way about our boys as being
" difficult." Let me now attempt to describe somewhat more
accurately, what kind of boy it is that comes to Barns.

First, as to age. Boys are admitted between the ages of nine and
twelve, and they normally stay (if the parents can be persuaded
to leave them) until school-leaving age.

We are pretty rigid about the upper age limit, because we do not
believe we can do very much with a boy in less than two years.
Sometimes, it is true, a remission of symptoms can be brought about
in far less than that time ; but a remission of symptoms is a rather
negative kind of achievement, and even if that were our only aim,
we should want to feel that the remission was not a temporary one.
We want so to build up a boy's character that we can see positive
traits taking the place of the negative ones, and to feel that he will
no longer need to display his symptoms even when he returns to his
old environment. Stephen Baillie is an example of the sort of thing
that is liable to happen. A bright, intelligent boy (I.Q. 98*), he
soon shewed himself an accomplished and invincible liar and a very
smart little pilferer, with a charming suavity of manner when he
was not in one of his " paddies." He came to us, let us say, in July,
1940. By February, 1941, I was able to remark in my case notes
that Stevie's symptoms seemed to have gone entirely. He was
happy, purposeful, and all that could be wished for, and we looked
forward to a nice long period of stabilisation for him. Then in
March he seemed to collapse completely. I will not go into the
case in detail as I expect to refer to it again in another context,
but his relapse followed some news from home which his mother
brought. We started all over again, but it was a rather more
stubborn job this time. However, by the Spring of 1942—a year
later—all was well and Stevie was his own man again. " Now,"
we said to ourselves, in our innocence and complacency, " There
can hardly be another situation like last year's to set him back again.
From now on it is Steadily Forward for Stevie." Four months

* An explanation of this term is given on page 28.

27

later (July, 1942), his mother, in spite of all my supplications and expostulations, took him home. By September she was beginning to take soundings concerning the possibility of his return ; at the end of the year she definitely broached the subject, and by February, 1943, he was back—his mother having given a solemn undertaking that this time there was to be no more taking away. We made another fresh start—symptoms as before, but the boy much more reserved and un-getatable. Four months later he was gone again —this time on his father's orders. I gave the father the most earnest warning that if Stevie were taken from us he would (in the father's own phrase) " take to a life of crime," and follow his elder brother to an Approved School—or worse. Time will shew whether I am right. Several such prognostications made in similar circumstances have unhappily been justified, but perhaps we shall be vouchsafed a miracle for Stevie. I hope so.

So there must be time for stabilisation, and for a positive building-up of defences against the home environment. As we cannot hope to do that in less than two years we do not take boys who are over the age of twelve. I know that other Hostels have a much quicker turn-over and I have recently been reading an account of a very well-conducted place where six to twelve months seems to be the average stay before a child is rebilleted or returned to its parents.* But if the children and the homes are anything like ours, I am very sceptical about the ultimate outcome.

The lower age limit, however, of nine, we keep fairly elastic, so that at any one time we may have boys of all ages from 8 to 14. The average age at present is 11.

Mental age, however, presents a very different picture and we found at one time that we were getting such a preponderance of dull boys that we had to say we would not accept more than a certain proportion of such boys. We expect the proportion of dull boys in a place like Barns to be fairly high, but not so high as it was at that time becoming.

In discussing Mental Ages it is convenient to use the device of the Intelligent Quotient, as this gives the relation of the Mental Age to the Chronological age (and thus the child's intellectual capacity) without the need to quote both every time. The term I.Q. is in these days fairly widely understood. If a child's intelligence has developed to the degree that is normally to be expected at his age ; if, that is to say, his Mental Age (M.A.) is equal to his Chronological Age (C.A.) ; he is said to have an I.Q. of 100. A child's I.Q. is proportionately higher or lower than 100 according to whether

* " Evacuation in Scotland," page 170 *et seq.*

his Mental Age is higher or lower than his Chronological Age. Thus, if a boy of ten years of age has only the intelligence to be expected of a boy of nine, he is said to have an I.Q. of 90 $\left(\dfrac{MA}{CA} \times 100\right)$.

A person's I.Q. is normally constant, whatever his age. People with an I.Q. lower than 70 are generally regarded as being certifiably mentally deficient, so that none of these come to Barns. The so-called ' dull and backward ' group have I.Q.'s between 70 and 85. The method by which a Mental Age is arrived at is not relevant to this discussion—there are excellent books on Mental Testing.

The distribution of intelligence among the general population follows roughly the curve of normal frequency. That is to say, about half the population are in the ' normal ' group of 90 to 110 I.Q., the number in each group above and below the normal being progressively fewer. For the purpose of comparison, however, it might be helpful to use a graph, drawn by Miss A. M. MacMeeken* of the I.Q.'s of schoolboys of about the Barns age, in four Scottish Cities which, with her permission, I append.

INTELLIGENCE OF SCHOOLBOYS IN FOUR SCOTTISH CITIES

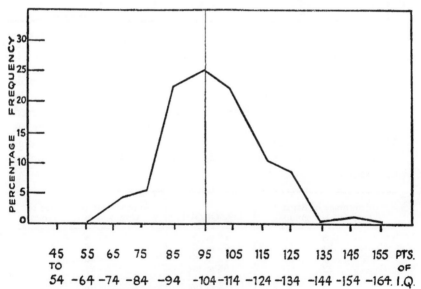

* See " The Intelligence, of a Representative Group of Scottish Schoolchildren," by A. M. MacMeeken, M.A. B.Ed. London University Press 1939.

It will be seen that there is not a great deal of difference between the number of boys with I.Q.'s above 100 and the number with I.Q.'s below. For the purpose of comparison, I reproduce the same graph, with a dotted line superimposed, to represent the incidence of the different I.Q.'s among Barns boys. It speaks for itself, but for greater clarity I have introduced (on both graphs) a median line which does not appear in the original.

INTELLIGENCE OF BARNS BOYS COMPARED WITH GENERAL
SCHOOLBOY POPULATION IN FOUR SCOTTISH CITIES

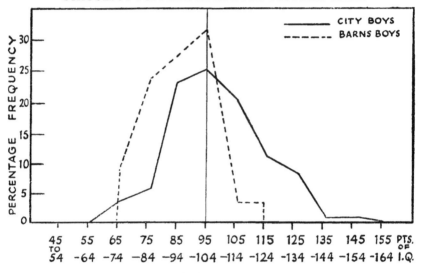

For those who prefer a tabular to a graphic statement, the table below gives I.Q. distributions at Barns in the first column, and in the third, the *approximate* distribution among the City boys referred to in the graph. These percentages are approximate, however, as Miss MacMeeken's tables are not arranged in the same groupings as her graph, and I have, therefore, taken the liberty of deducing the percentages from the graph.

Percentage of Barns boys in each group.	I.Q. GROUP.	Approximate percentage of City boys in each group.
8	65 to 74	4
24	75 to 84	6
28	85 to 94	23
32	95 to 104	25
4	105 to 114	20
2	115 to 124	10
0	125 to 134	8

When we add to these figures the fact that some of the low I.Q.'s are among the young boys and some of the high among the oldest, we find that we have to deal with boys whose Mental Ages range from about six to about sixteen. It will be seen, however, that most of our boys are in the lower reaches of the normal or the higher reaches of the sub-normal group, and that a highly intelligent boy is rather a rarity.

When we come to examine the *educational* status of the boys, the picture becomes even blacker. I will merely say at this point that most of the boys have on admission an educational attainment well below the normal for their years and—what is much more significant—many of them have an educational standard well below what is to be expected at their *mental* age. But a fuller discussion of this factor will be found in Chapter 11, which deals with the school.

So much for ages, chronological, mental and educational. I give it for what it is worth. There is a value in the reckoning of I.Q.'s and administering of Attainments Tests and so forth, and I should not like to underestimate it. But it is possible to overestimate it.

I like very much the distinction which I am told the Anthroposophists make between " heart " intelligence and " head " intelligence*. Intelligence tests only measure head intelligence. There is no way of measuring the other kind, though it is not difficult to recognise when it is present. The President to whom I referred at the beginning of this book did not have a very high I.Q. and his educational attainments were shocking. But he will " get by " in the test of living with a comfortable margin, unless I am much in error, because he is well-endowed with heart intelligence. You couldn't beat him for pacifying a recalcitrant rebel, or consoling someone who felt irremediably injured. At the hearing of charges, too, he displayed the wisdom of Solomon. An example occurred only the other day. Wyn Stoddard charged someone who had been making a mess in the dormitory just after it had been cleaned, by burning bits of paper in it. The Committee was stumped, but not so the President. " Archie has made extra work for the cleaning staff, so he ought to do some work for them. He seems fond of burning paper. All right, let him collect all the bits of paper that are lying about outside, and burn them." Thus society's protest was made, restitution effected, a penalty imposed, and a lovely bonfire to end up with. Could the most intellectual

* Are these perhaps the " Raison Sensitive " and " Raison Intellectuelle " of Rousseau ?

of stipendiaries more happily mete out justice ?   Or there is Leslie
Dorking. His I.Q. is 93. Not very low, perhaps, but his educational
attainment was much lower.   He was chronically and (apparently)
incurably lethargic and tardy ; his nose was always running ; he
wet his bed nearly every night, and he fouled his trousers regularly.
Altogether a nasty, dull, dirty oaf you might think.   But he was
never happier than when listening to music or poetry.   For poetry
indeed, he had an almost inexhaustible appetite, and would listen
with his eyes sparkling for as long as one cared to read.   That
is the sort of thing I imagine the Anthroposophists to mean by
heart intelligence.   I hope they will forgive me if I've got the
wrong idea.   But if it isn't what they mean, it is what I mean, and
there's lots of it to be found among Barns boys.   Incidentally, if I
may digress, Leslie serves as a warning against becoming too
involved in high falutin psychology.   We discussed his lumpish-
ness, his nose running and all the other unpleasant things at Staff
meetings and made impressive sounding notes about " weeping
diathesis," but he got no better.   Indeed, he got worse.   Then
one day I was giving the boys their weekly Hygiene lesson, when
it suddenly occurred to me that we might do worse than try
the effect of a nasal douche on Leslie.   I will not say it cured
him the next day.   But after a couple of months of douching
Leslie was a different character, his nasty symptoms near to
disappearing point, and he skittish to the point of being a positive
nuisance.

So much then, as I believe I said, for age and mental status.
Let us go on now to look at the background from which the boys
come.

They are all Edinburgh boys, and they all (or nearly all) come
from working-class families, generally from poor working-class
families.   This usually means that they have lived in one of those
tall and gloomy tenement houses about the High Street or Leith
Walk, though a few of them come from one of the Housing
Estates.

In most cases there is something amiss in the family relationships.
All writers on the subject of juvenile delinquency have noticed the
monotonous and tragic regularity with which this factor appears.
I have nothing novel to say about it ; I merely add my little pebble
to the enormous heap.

Before we can discuss the incidence of this factor among Barns
boys I had better say what I mean by " something amiss " in the
family relationships.   The ideal family is one where there
is a mother and a father who are in love and married to

each other*, and who are fond of their children. As there is often no way of knowing whether parents are " in love " or not, I shall content myself with regarding a family as normal if there are two parents who seem to be fond of their children and between whom there is not obvious and chronic discord.

But there are very many ways in which a child may be denied even these limited requirements. The child may be illegitimate and may not know one parent or both parents ; one or both parents may have died or deserted ; the parents may be divorced or living apart ; they may be living together in a state of mutual antagonism. I have never come across a case of parents being fond of each other but not of the children, but all the phenomena I have listed are to be found among the parents of Barns boys except that there is no case of both parents having died. Of the fifty boys whose I.Q.'s I gave above (fifty is a convenient number for calculating percentages and we haven't had a hundred yet) only four per cent. are known to fulfill my modest requirements for normality—and those two boys are brothers ! We know that seventy-two per cent. of these boys come from families where there are present one or more of the factors of inadequacy that I have given. In a further 18 per cent. some measure of abnormality is strongly suspected though not proved ; and about the remaining six per cent. we have no information. I should, perhaps, add that in compiling these figures I have ignored separations of parents that are due solely to war circumstances, such as the father being in one of the Forces. I do not know what is the incidence of these factors in the general population, but I am not writing a scientific treatise, and we are all sufficiently familiar with the general population to be able to guess that at any rate more than ten per cent. are normal in the sense that I am using the word. Dr. Cyril Burt†, writing twenty years ago, gave " defective family relationships " as present in 57.9 per cent. of his delinquent cases, and 25.7 per cent. of his non-delinquent, but of course his criteria are not identical with mine, and he is speaking of a much more numerous group.

Some of the parents take very little interest in their children, some (though this is much the smaller number) fuss over them unduly. Some boys do not seem to get even so much as a birthday card from one year's end to the next, though even in these cases one

---

* I do not wish to suggest that it is impossible for parents to love each other and their children without having gone through a form of marriage. But as Society is at present constituted the stigma of illegitimacy may have a grave effect on a child's development, socially and psychologically, however excellent the parents.

† " The Young Delinquent," page 53.

c

never knows when the parent may be seized with an attack of conscience and suddenly turn up at Barns bearing gifts, or making up for a year's neglect by taking the boy home again. Though I think it only fair to add that often a parent's failure to write may be due as much as anything to general inarticulateness and semi-illiteracy. I do not know whether, among all the other plans that are being discussed for that millenial post-war period anyone is thinking of making an assessment of the results of half a century of compulsory education. I suspect that the investigators would get as great a shock as some of our respectable country cousins got when our city children were evacuated on to them ! However, that is more or less beside my point, and in any case this chapter is supposed to be a mere statement of facts rather than of comment.

Next, then, for the question which so often infuriates me when it falls from the all too audible lips of the casual and curious visitor— " What is *he* here for ? " The answer to that question is of course, that he is here because he is unhappy and at odds with Society ; we want to help him to find a way to be happy and to find a constructive expression of his rebelliousness. " I am not concerned with making good little citizens," said Russell Hoare, of Riverside Village (I quote from memory) ; " I am out to make rebels." Well—we don't need to do that at Barns ; they are pretty good little rebels when they come to hand, many of them. But we do want to see to it that their rebelliousness means something, and is not merely a futile and painful kicking against the pricks.

But, of course, our visitor really didn't mean that. He meant, " What was the particular manifestation of the boy's unhappiness that caused some concerned adult to say : ' This boy had better go to Barns ' ? " What are the symptoms complained of ?

Perhaps this question is best answered by means of another table, using again the fifty boys about whom other figures were given. We usually find when a boy has been with us for a little while that there are other symptoms besides those mentioned by the referring agency, and I have, therefore, made two columns, one for the " Referral Symptoms " and one for " Subsequent Symptoms," though subsequent may mean discovered subsequently or developed subsequently. Some boys, *e.g.*, are bed-wetters before they come, but we are left to find that out after the boy gets here ; others start bed-wetting after they reach Barns, but both these would come in the second column.

SYMPTOM.	Number reported on referral	Number discovered subsequently	TOTALS
Stealing ; " dishonesty " ; Housebreaking	22	9	31
* Enuresis ; † Encopresis ; " dirty habits "	5	16	21
Truancy	16	0	16
" Unmanageable " ; " Wild " ; " Self-willed " ; " Beyond control "	14	0	14
General insecurity picture-aggressiveness, irrational fears, &c.	2	12	14
Temper Tantrums	3	10	13
Lying	3	4	7
Speech Defects	1	3	4
Wandering	4	0	4
Destructiveness	1	2	3
Backward ; Ineducable	2	0	2
Cruelty	2	0	2
Tardiness	2	0	2
Begging	1	0	1
Indecency	1	0	1
TOTALS	79	56	135

* Incontinence of urine.
† Incontinence of fæces.

There is here an accumulation of 135 symptoms distributed among fifty boys, and you might assume, therefore, that everything has been here recorded that could possibly be described as a symptom. That is not the case at all. The symptoms shewn are all what might fairly be described as *major* symptoms, any one of which would call for special treatment, though they are not necessarily all symptoms which, taken by themselves, would have justified a boy being sent to Barns. I confess that in compiling the list of symptoms it was in some cases difficult to know where to draw the line. In the case, for example, of " backwardness." Only two boys were referred to us for this cause, but as I have already said, the majority of the boys are more or less backward on arrival, many of them seriously so. This I have simply ignored. Lying again is difficult. We have no George Washingtons at Barns, but there are some boys who are clearly more outstanding liars than others, and these are duly recorded. Then there is a factor to which I have made no reference at all, merely because our figures are incomplete. That is the factor of what is known as " laterality." Most of us are right-handed and right-eyed, but some, who may be called left-lateral, are left-handed or left-eyed or both, and it has been shewn that the presence of this factor will probably make for considerable difficulty in learning and may also lead to behaviour difficulties*. Dr. M. MacMeeken came to Barns one day and very kindly applied her laterality tests to the 28 boys then present. It was found that 16 of the 28 were left-handed or left-eyed or both, and that six others displayed other characteristics connected with abnormal laterality. Finally, I have made no reference to the two boys whom I believe to be pre-psychotics, because it ill-becomes the layman to rush in where doctors fear to tread.

It will be seen then that in seriousness of character difficulty, the boy who comes to Barns is very much akin to the sort of boy who goes to the Approved School, and there is very little doubt that, but for the war and the consequent accident of our half-way house being available, that is where many of them would have gone. Seventeen of the fifty are definitely known to have had Court experience, and three are now in Approved Schools.

There are two other questions, of a factual nature that I am often asked. When I have answered them I shall feel that I have described the material adequately enough and, with a sigh of relief in which I invite the reader to share, we can pass on to the method.

My penultimate point then is the referring agency. Technically, our boys are supposed to come from other billets in the Edinburgh Reception Areas (*i.e.*, areas to which Edinburgh children are evacuated) on the complaint of hostesses to Billeting Officers. Of the fifty boys I have been dealing with here, only thirteen came to us in this way, and the proportion has since become smaller. More usually they come direct from Edinburgh, being evacuated straight to Barns. In every case they must come through the Edinburgh Evacuation Officer who, very conveniently, is also the City Education Officer. Most of the boys come to us on the direct recommendation and at the wish of the Education Authority, it being understood that the decision as to whether any given boy is suitable for treatment at Barns rests with me. Schoolmasters sometimes complain about a boy's behaviour, or there may be complaints from parents; sometimes it is the School Attendance Officer who initiates the plan to send a boy to Barns; sometimes the suggestion may be made at the Court, when proceedings are dropped on the understanding that the boy is to be evacuated. In all these cases application is made to the Evacuation Officer for the boy's evacuation, the suggestion at the same time being made that he come to Barns. But there are also private as distinct from public agencies that want to send boys to Barns—Child Guidance

---

* See " Developmental Aphasia in Educationally Retarded Children," by M. MacMeeken, M.A., B.Ed., Ph.D., London University Press.

Clinics, Social workers, Church workers, and so forth. A small proportion of our boys have come from such sources, though here again the referring agency must work through the ordinary evacuation channels. During the last twelve months, the Edinburgh Corporation has set up its own Child Guidance Clinic, and it is now usual for boys to come through the clinic.

Finally, we must look at the question of the duration of treatment and the causes of its termination.

If ever the flame of our enthusiasm flickers—and flicker it sometimes does—that flicker is caused by a draught from this direction more often than from all other directions combined. The difficulty of keeping boys until we have finished with them has militated against success more than any other single cause ; more indeed, than all other causes put together, if we except those arising from our own human frailty. It has been our one great bugbear, and the effort to combat it has consumed time, energy, skill and patience that should have been spent in the service of more constructive ends.

Barns is part of the Evacuation Scheme. Evacuation is not compulsory, and children may be taken home again for the most frivolous of reasons, or for no reason at all. That is what has happened at Barns.

Absconding we do not mind. It is one of the legitimate risks of the trade, and we should be much surprised if it did not happen. It is merely a symptom of the unhappy child's desire to escape from himself—and he usually comes back.

What irritates, alarms, and finally exasperates us is the completely irresponsible attitude of so many of the parents. Boys are taken home—quite irrespective of the progress of treatment, and often with profuse thanks for ' all you have done for him '—because a brother is coming home from some other place ; because the parents have been asked to supply a pair of boots (though this is never *given* as the reason) ; because ' his father has decided to have him home ' ; because the parents have moved into a new house ; because the parents have separated—or have come together again—or re-married ; because someone is needed to mind the baby, or run the errands. Sometimes our earnest beseechings and supplications are not without effect, but sometimes parents are quite deaf to reason or entreaty, and after listening to a long, and sometimes an impassioned appeal, they will stolidly reply " Aye, well, I think I'll have him home." The following, though an exceptional letter, is still typical of the attitude which is blind to the needs of the boy and sees only the comfort and convenience of the parents. The boy in question had a very bad record, and I shall be surprised if he is not by this time in an Approved School. He had been at

Barns three days when this letter arrived . . . " Mr. Willis. I want my boy Clothes packed up and send him home with his brother, as I can't sleep at night thinking about him as he is the only one out of the house if his Father had not been working he would have been out for him today it is fair knocking me up and I can't stand the strain any longer."

How often have I, in moments of exasperation, fervently agreed with that alleged saying of Mr. Punch—that the very last people who ever ought to be allowed to have children are parents !

It is difficult to give a real picture of how long the boys stay with us, because obviously, we cannot include those who are still at Barns as we do not know how long they are going to stay, and some of them have already been with us longer than any who have left. Bearing this saving clause in mind then, I will confine myself to the boys who have so far left Barns, and they are 46 in number. Three of these I will exclude. They left because they got into trouble with the police while they were at Barns. One went straight to an Approved School, after having been with us a year ; the other two (who burgled the Head teacher's cottage, *see page* 22), left at my suggestion, because I thought that the fact of their being no longer resident in the neighbourhood might help them when they " came up." In this I maligned the Court, which is as enlightened and conscientious a Children's Court as any I have ever had dealings with. These two boys had been with us about two years, and, incidentally, both did eventually get to an Approved School. Excluding then these three boys as being in a special category, there have been 43 " leavers," and these can be divided into two groups—those who left without our approval and against advice, and those of whose departure we were more or less able to approve. The former category is the larger, containing no fewer than thirty boys. I will not burden you with a catalogue of the reasons given for their removal—you have had a few examples above. I will merely tabulate how long they stayed, mentioning in passing that two left because they simply refused to stay.

Of these 30 " unsatisfactory leavers " then :

6 stayed for 1 month or less,	5 stayed for 13 to 18 months,
4 stayed for 1 to 6 months,	4 stayed for 19 to 24 months,
7 stayed for 7 to 12 months,	4 stayed for 25 to 30 months.

Four of these thirty boys have since been admitted to Approved Schools ; and one to an Institution for the Mentally Defective. Two have been prosecuted for petty offences without serious consequence. Judged by the negative standard of not having got into trouble, the other 20 seem to be all right.

Then there are the 13 " satisfactory leavers." None of these was with us for less than 6 months.

3 stayed for 7 to 12 months,	3 stayed for 25 to 30 months,
2 stayed for 13 to 18 months,	2 stayed for 31 to 36 months,
1 stayed for 19 to 24 months,	1 stayed for 37 to 40 months,

1 had two spells of 18 and 12 months respectively.

The three boys who were with us less than a year never seemed to us to have been very difficult, and were therefore rebilleted. One boy was returned home while still of school age as being " sufficiently improved " (in the opinion of his parents, Wills reluctantly assenting) and the others all left on reaching—or just before reaching—school-leaving age. Two of these we should perhaps have preferred to keep a little longer and significantly they are the only two who have so far given serious cause for anxiety, but under the watchful eye of our Social Worker they seem now to be getting over their difficulties. Five of these boys went to jobs found by us, two to suitable jobs, and two to less suitable jobs, found by their parents.

I give these figures for what they are worth, which, I fear is very little. We could if we wished, make the facile boast that none of those who stayed with us as long as we wished has since got into trouble—but they are very few, and there is still plenty of time ! Then a boy may have been improved tremendously ; he may be a changed character exuding all the virtues and yet he may, by an unfortunate conjunction of circumstances, commit an offence and thus be listed a " failure." On the other hand, a boy may be little improved, but may just manage, by luck more than by judgment, to avoid the clutch of the policeman, and thus be considered a " success." Even those who left against our advice seem in some cases to have been very much helped, and in some cases, apparently, completely tided over their difficulties by their stay with us. But even if it were possible to assess results, which it is not, it is much too soon to do so. In five year's time, perhaps . . . ?

It will seem to many arrogant and stupid, but it is my firm conviction that the results are not of fundamental importance in the consideration of the method. If the results are poor, that will shew that the method has been faultily applied which, God knows, we realise already. It will not invalidate the method.

But you will be impatient to know what this method is, in which I have such sublime confidence. Let us abandon these deceptive facts and figures, and get on with the theory.

CHAPTER FOUR

SHARING RESPONSIBILITIES

" . . . there are two ways of contesting, the one by law, the other by force ;
the first method is proper to men, the second to beasts."
                                        MACHIAVELLI—" The Prince."

FOR a few weeks before Barns was quite ready to receive its permanent guests, it was used for another purpose. The war seemed to have been on a long time then—nearly a whole year in fact—and evacuation hostesses were getting a little tired of their guests. So it was arranged that we should take batches of boys (rarely more than half-a-dozen at a time) for a week or two's stay at Barns, to give them a holiday and their hostesses a rest. I suppose a couple of dozen boys must have enjoyed this privilege during July and August, 1940.

Such nice boys they were! Polite, gentlemanly, obedient, respectful, considerate, spineless, inert, thoroughly devoid of initiative and as dull as a war-time dinner. They took it as a matter of course that they must not go near the river or play with the water and they would not have dreamed of venturing down the drive unless officially conducted by an adult. Their insufferable docility had brought us somewhere near screaming point when the first batch of permanent Barns boys arrived. I will not say that we have never since cast for a moment a regretful eye on the peaceful days of that halcyon summer ; but never for more than a moment, and we rejoiced in being, at last, surrounded by boys of spirit. *These* boys were not afraid to venture down the drive ! On the contrary, the first thing they did was—like sensible animals —to find their bearings. It is true that they had heard of some kind of school that they were expected to attend, and they knew from experience (their pre-Barns experience) that the penalty for truanting was a good belting, but that was neither here nor there— they must take a look at the country. And so they did. Without respect for boundaries or fences, or owners' rights, they proceeded to make themselves familiar with the countryside. One fresh batch after another did the same thing—we came to look upon it as inevitable that new boys would skip school once or twice during the first week in order to take a look round. I well remember the first occasion—or rather the report of it, for I was not present. We had six boys, and five of them went off for a walk just before school was due to start. Kenneth Roberton went to look for them on his bike and in due course found them. They were quite unabashed. They were truanting and everyone knows you get the belt for that. All right. It was a fair cop. Kenneth was wearing an admirable belt, and they suggested that he took it off and extracted suitable payment for a morning off, after which he and they could go each their several ways. They *were* abashed, however, when Kenneth said that was not his plan at all. He had come to take them back because the teacher didn't like the idea of having one boy instead of six ; and back eventually they went. That was not the last time any of these boys truanted and—believe it or not—we did not finally have an end to truanting until Ben took over the school, and it was perfectly clear to everyone that there was no question of punishment or even a punitive attitude to "skipping school." That, however, is beside the present point. What I was leading up to was not truanting but trespassing. There are no neat little notices saying " keep off the grass " in the fields around Barns so the presumption—to a city boy—is that you may go on it—and anyway, " There's naeb'dy looking." This was one of our first difficulties and a very early matter for discussion at a meeting of everybody, which we called a House meeting.

It was at the second meeting that " David Wills explained why Lord Wemyss didn't want us to go over the fences and we all agreed not to do it." The very next week the question came up again—I had received a complaint from a neighbour that the boys had climbed a fence and upset a hay-cock—" Kenneth then told how he had been up to Haswellsykes to see the farmer and apologise. The farmer was upset about it because a haycock is worth £4, and if it is upset so that the rain gets in it is worth nothing. But he was very decent about it so Kenneth thought we ought to be decent to him in return and keep our promise not to go over the fences "—and the names of those who had already broken their promise were recorded for future reference. So the attitude to trespassing gradually stiffened until one day Billy Bell was told that he was not to go outside the precincts of Barns unless accompanied by an adult, because he seemed quite incapable of preventing himself going to places where he should not be. Later still, it became the practice to make a list every Friday of those who were considered capable of walking abroad without trespassing and they were called " Freemen "—the others were not allowed away from Barns unless an adult took them.

I was sorry in a way that we had all this fuss about trespassing, because I have myself very little conscience in the matter, and yet

I had to set myself deliberately to build up a public opinion against it, which is a thing I very much object to doing. Except during birds-nesting time (when the sanctity of game-woods is apt to be violated) we have very little trouble about trespassing now, not only because of the tradition which has been set up, but because it is a question which does not arise. A trespasser is merely a stranger. " Trespassers will be prosecuted " only means, as a rule " Anyone I don't know will be prosecuted if he steps on my land." Our boys have made themselves familiar to one of our neighbours at least, and he now never complains about them being on his land unless they are being a nuisance. Indeed, all along our chief trouble has been not the farmers but the gamekeeper, but that is a long story and perhaps an irrelevant one.

I had to establish, by the pressure of my influence, an attitude against trespassing because the farmers as well as the shooters are all tenants of the people who so kindly lent us the house, so I could not risk too much trouble with them. Normally, the method is to allow rules and traditions to come into being as a result of experience, but in this matter I explained my position quite candidly and I think they understood it. I told them that in most institutions of this kind they wouldn't get a chance to go out unaccompanied. Here they were free, the price of freedom was eternal vigilance, and as our neighbours were in a position to put the screw on us, we'd better be pretty vigilant. Then I saw to it that whenever there was any trespassing the matter was brought up, instead of waiting (as I should in most other matters) until the failure to raise the matter had brought its inevitable unfortunate consequences.

In this matter then—and in some others concerning our relations with outsiders—I have deliberately " worked on " the boys. In general I have been more ready to run risks inside the house than outside, because if a boy makes a slip outside—and gets caught— we are liable to lose him to an Approved School. That is one of the advantages that an Approved School has over Barns—they are much less likely to lose any boy who abuses his freedom than we are.

There are three grades of authority at Barns. There is the authority of the adults, which is absolute on matters of health, and which includes the delegated authority of outside agencies, such as the Education Authority ; there is the " influence " which I deliberately bring to bear (as infrequently as possible), usually in connection with something concerning our relations with the outside world—less often to prevent a boy being victimised ; and then there is the authority of the House meeting (now known as the General Meeting), which covers everything else. We try to avoid the hypocrisy of saying " The boys make all the rules," and then expecting them to make only the rules *we* want to see made. Where a clear law must be laid down, the adults lay it down and no monkey business. We (the Staff) lay down the bed-times, we made the rule " No bathing except under adult supervision." We explain the reasons for these rules, but we are not so dishonest as to explain the need for a rule and then say, " So shall we make a rule about it ? " when we know perfectly well that a rule must be made whether the meeting wants to make one or not. Outside authority says (in effect) " You must go to school," and although we should, on the whole, prefer voluntary lessons, Authority relies on the adults to see that their order is obeyed. But although adults or outside authority make some rules, the enforcement of those rules has usually been taken on by the democratic governing machinery of the House. And because we have always been perfectly honest about what matters were, and what were not, within the jurisdiction of the Meeting, we have never had to deal with the grouse which I believe is not uncommon in some " self-governing " schools. "We're supposed to be self-governing—why can't we please ourselves " about this or that. In fact, we rarely use the phrase " self-government " because it is not self-government, and I very much oubt whether there is any school where—if the adults are quite honest with themselves—there is complete self-government.

Where, then, there is no choice, the adults make the law ; where there *is* a choice, the meeting makes it. True, the adults have a right to attend meetings, say their say, and use their votes, but in practice we try not to influence a decision unless, as I have said, it is something which concerns our relations with the outside world, or something which is likely to affect vitally a boy's happiness. Even when we do that, we are most careful to see that the boys understand the justice and rightness of the course we favour— indeed if we do not, the voting will go against us. That is another reason that we are sparing with adult influence. If it begins to be suspected that adults are influencing too many decisions, the time will come when any course recommended by an adult will be voted against, just for that reason. Indeed, that happened at our very first meeting when—as everyone was new—it was taken for granted that anything suggested by an adult was suggested with some ulterior motive, and should, therefore, be voted against. It was over the question of orderly duties. I explained that paid adults had been appointed to do most of the housework, but there were various jobs which no-one was paid to do, and for which we should have to make arrangements between us. Those jobs were bed-making, dish-washing and potato peeling, and I asked how they were to be done. As at first no suggestions seemed forthcoming, and as I have had a great deal of experience of arranging orderly duties, I put forward a scheme . . . " but Bruce Cobber said he had a better idea . . . After a lot of talk we decided to have Bruce's idea, beginning next Sunday." This was not the last time that orderly duties were discussed, and that last time is not yet. A few weeks ago, someone got the idea that the system then in operation let off the staff too lightly, so another scheme (the nth) was devised which seemed to achieve the objective of making it rather harder for the adults. Since it involved the adults all working together (instead of being distributed among the boys), it also made things much harder for everyone else ! But never mind—the adults aren't getting away with anything ! I have explained that the new scheme is much easier for the staff, but the boys think that is just sour grapes.

At the early House meetings I was self-appointed Chairman and Secretary, but after a few weeks, when we had begun to fill up, I said it was time the meeting chose its own officers. So they elected me as Chairman, my wife as Secretary, and Kenneth Roberton as Treasurer ! Such timidity astonished me, but I let it pass—I knew it would not last long and I insisted that the term of office should be for one month only. As a matter of fact this timidity (which I hasten to add, expressed itself in no other aspect of the life of the establishment) lasted longer than I expected, and although they rang the changes among the adults, it was not until three months had passed that they elected a boy as Chairman— Gilbert Rivers—with myself as Secretary. The final minute on that occasion reads " Jacob Everson said he would not obey the instructions of the new Chairman, so it was decided he should not attend School meetings." Jacob (though none of us suspected this at the time) was to become one of our most distinguished chair-men, and his name stands out in the annals of Barns like a Cecil or a Chatham or a Churchill in the history of England. Two weeks later we read " Jacob Everson sent a request that he be permitted to attend House meetings in future. He was brought into the meeting and asked whether he was ready to promise to obey the Chairman in future. He said he was, so he was allowed to attend meetings again."

As one looks through the minutes, they give the impression of having been very orderly, well-conducted meetings. But it is a profoundly misleading impression. The minutes record merely decisions, with, perhaps, a few notes describing how the decision was arrived at. Disorder is not usually recorded, but there was plenty of it, and we do occasionally find an entry like this—on 9.12.40—" After this, the meeting became disorderly and David (I was Chairman then) dismissed it." What the Secretary meant was that after " that " (whatever that may have been) the meeting became just *too* disorderly, and it was impossible to carry on.

So we went on from week to week, arranging and re-arranging the orderly duties, discussing the care of the games equipment, talking about trespassing, arranging parties and concerts, arguing about the inter-dormitory competition we had in those days, appointing a Committee to buy a vase for the post-mistress, in return for the sweets she sent us from time to time—and so on. There were also very many items of this kind :—" Molly (cook) reminded us of the possible consequences of playing about with the food lift. There was a lot of talk about this, but no definite decision was made " . . . " David Wills raised the question of the electric light bulbs that were missing, but everyone said they knew nothing about it." . . . " The Chairman complained that on certain evenings when painting and handwork were being carried on, boys were in the habit of disturbing these quiet indoor activities by careering through the house, slamming doors. Bobbie Dodd suggested that these boys go outside or stay in the play-room. Chairman suggested that one night might be set aside for chasing. Wally Straight suggested that there should be no chasing while indoor activities were being carried on, and this was carried, with the proviso that Tuesday evenings and Sunday afternoons should be reserved for chasing about the house " . . . and so on.

It was one thing to make all these rules and prohibitions, but it was quite another to see that they were kept, and before long this became one of the principal pre-occupations of the meeting. There was not only a matter of seeing that *Statute* Law, as we may perhaps describe it, was carried out ; there was also the question of what, on the same analogy, we may describe as Common Law (and even, after a time, something very much like Case Law). We have no rule in the minute book forbidding stealing, and for a long time there was none prohibiting assault. But they, and many such thing, are by common consent regarded as improper, and there were many boys seeking redress and protection. All such cases came before the House meeting and indeed they took up most of the time. We therefore set up, eventually, a committee to deal with charges. It consisted of one boy from each dormitory (five in all) and one adult, and it met more or less every day.

I regard this Court (for so we may regard it, though it has never had that name) as one of the most important aspects of shared responsibility. In any community—whether of children or of adults—there is (or usually has been so far in the history of man) a tendency, however slight, for the strong to exploit the weak, and it is necessary to have some form of protection against this. Most schools have their bullies, and in the orthodox school they often have a pretty free hand. A boy who appeals for adult aid against the aggressor is considered a cissie, and not only by the other boys ! In any case, the chances are that after he has sought aid he will get a worse pummelling than ever for being a sneak. We have all read the autobiographies of sensitive boys who have endured the privilege of a Public School Education, and although there are perhaps not so many autobiographies of Elementary School boys, I can assure my readers (for I was one) that it is just about as bad there. But I will resist the temptation to anticipate a chapter of my own autobiography, enlightening though it might be, in this context. Our Court does come, I believe, as near to solving this problem as it is possible to come short of curing the bullies—a process which is being carried on at the same time by other agencies than the Court. In the first place, if a boy brings a charge to the Committee he is not sneaking—or clyping, as they say in Scotland. A clype is a boy who crawls up to some adult and surreptitiously whispers his tale of woe into his ear. Bringing a charge to the Committee is no more clyping than is calling in the police if your house is robbed. That is clearly understood and accepted by all—so charges are brought. (We sometimes have over a hundred in one week !) Where restitution or compensation can be ordered, that is the usual course. If " A " steals " B's " toffee, he is made to replace it. If " B " breaks " C's " roller skate he is ordered to get it mended (he may have to ask an adult to do it for him, but that is neither here not there—he gets the damage repaired) ; " C " has knocked over the " gang-hut " that " D " has spent several days constructing, and is ordered to build it up again. " Och, never mind," says " D," " I'll build it ma sel'." He realises suddenly that most of the fun of the " gang-hut " was in the building, and he doesn't want to give " C " that pleasure ! But—and here is the important point—he is quite satisfied, and the breach is healed. Often there is very little the Committee can do, except to hear the case—both sides of the case—and express an opinion as to who is in the wrong. But equally often that is all that is needed. If the frustrated boy who has had something unpleasant done to him, feels that he can explain his situation to a sympathetic audience, receive a measure of condolence and be assured that he is in the right—that is all he needs, more often than not. If, on the other hand, he has to suffer the minor annoyances of some petty bully, or some merely thoughtless bigger boy, and be unable to do anything about it at all, he is liable to become warped and embittered and be continually whining. I have noticed repeatedly that a boy will come to the Committee boiling over with a sense of frustration and injustice, and leave the Committee perfectly happy, though nothing whatever has been done ! That is almost impossible in a normal school—it would be sneaking ! It is an everyday occurrence at Barns.

"But is it good for the boys not to learn to stand up for themselves?" some people ask. And sometimes a new boy will disdain to use the Court, saying "I can stick up for myself." There are two answers to this. One is that in seeking legal redress a boy *is* standing up for himself, and successfully, whereas very often the attempt to stand up for himself in the other way is the merest futility. The other reply is in the nature of a *tu quoque*, but is not without point. Do *you*, dear superior adult, always "stand up for yourself"? Or do you send for a policeman? One of the things which principally distinguishes civilised from savage society is the willingness of individuals to surrender the right to "stick up for themselves." When that right is equally surrendered by the nations . . . But I will not digress.

Even, however, in the cases where nothing seems to have been done except comfort the aggrieved party, something else has in fact been done, and often a very important something. Public opinion has been expressed. When the Headmaster stands before the School at assembly, and verbally castigates a boy or a set of boys, he may make a few people feel a little uncomfortable for a little while—perhaps for as long as he is speaking—but he is unlikely to have any permanent effect on the persons concerned. He is an adult, and adults have what seems to children, a cross-eyed view about pretty well everything, and after all the Old Man's paid to stand up there and make orations. Even if the castigations take place in private, the effect is pretty much the same, except that there is less chance of the victim feeling himself a bit of a hero. But if the other boys are heard to say, "That's a pretty lousy thing to do," the effect is totally different. This is an expression of real opinion, not another manifestation of adult prejudice. It goes home. Indeed, I find that very often the adult has to temper the wind a little to the shorn bully. On one occasion I was unable to do so. Martin Dodd was one of the first boys to come to Barns. He was the biggest of the bunch, and remained the biggest and the toughest for some time. At first he had it all his own way, and was indeed rather popular with some. Those with whom he was not very popular did not dare to say so, and pretended to admire everything he did. After a time it began to be realised that one could say what one really thought about boys of this kind, and some of the more courageous began to say it, although—in those early days—more than one got a bloody nose or a nasty kick on the shins for saying it. That, however, increased the anger of the population against Martin and the time came when he was so unpopular with the other boys that he ran away. His mother persuaded him to return, but he said he had only come for his things so I tried to use the " influence " to which I have referred earlier. I had a talk with Martin first, and tried to get him in a better mood, but without success. That failing, I had a talk with the other boys, tried to get a little sympathy for Martin, suggested that he had learnt his lesson and that we should now welcome him back and make it clear that we did not want him to leave. Then I made the dreadful mistake. I was perfectly confident that I had carried them with me, and therefore said (hoping to impress the boy), " Hands up those who want Martin to stay and have another go." To my horror and surprise only half-a-dozen or so put up their hands. This was the chance of the oppressed and bullied, and they took it. There was no keeping Martin after that, though I may add that it was only because I thought there was no hope of keeping him in the first place that I tried this method. I should, perhaps, add that this did not take place in Martin's presence. He is in an Approved School now, writes regularly, and visits us when he has a holiday. Here, Public Opinion was expressed too strongly, and that is why I say that one of our duties is to temper the wind sometimes. It has never happened since, and I doubt whether it will ever happen again. Unfortunate as it was, however, one cannot help feeling that it may have made Martin Dodd realise that people really do dislike bullying, and that it is not merely an adult prejudice. Not for one moment do I suggest that that will cure Martin of bullying ; but I do believe it will help him to try to " get a grip on himself."

I do not know whether I am deceiving myself by unconsciously fathering the thought on the wish, but it has always seemed to me that there was very little inclination to deal with these charges merely by the infliction of retributive punishment. It is true that in those days there was always an adult with non-punitive ideas present at the Committees, but even now, when the Committee meets as often as not without an adult, that still seems to be true. The aim generally was (and is) to try to find some way to avoid a repetition of the offence. Thus the limiting of the trespasser's

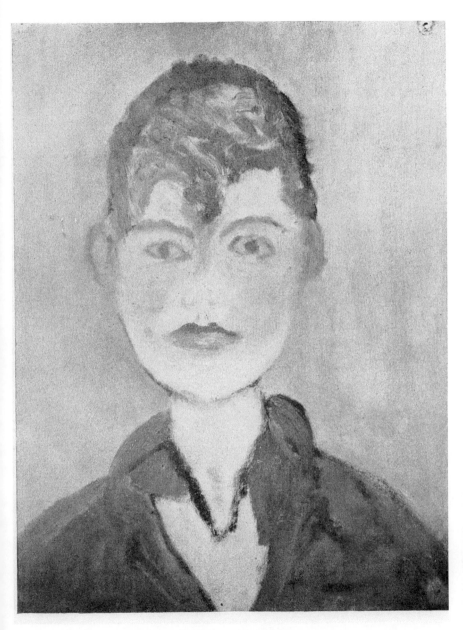

LESLIE DORKING
Self portrait

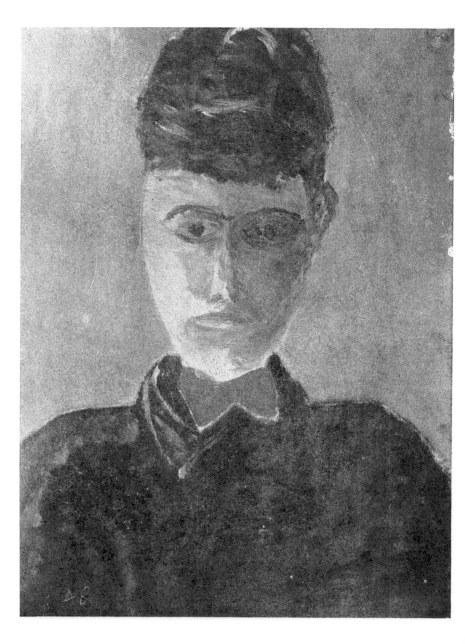

IAN BURNS
Self portrait

freedom, and the giving of a " keeper " to a boy who was always getting into trouble. Theft, as I have said, is usually dealt with by restitution or compensation, and the nearest approach to punishment has been in connection with assault. It began by Ian Burns being fined a halfpenny for hitting someone, later the fine was increased, and ultimately, the fine became a form of damages, in that it was given not to the Meeting funds, but to the person who had been assaulted. The point that I made, in expressing my preference for this way of dealing with it, was that " A " had done something unpleasant to " B," and he should now, therefore, compensate " B " by doing something pleasant to him.

We continued then in this sort of way—more or less rowdy weekly meetings, which everyone attended (or at least was entitled to attend), daily Committees, and the Staff taking a much more prominent place than really I thought we ought. Technically, there was freedom and a good deal of self-government, but meetings and decisions were rather " adult-ridden." Let it not be thought, however, that this meant that what was really happening was that everything was nice and orderly, and that in fact the adults were running the place behind a façade of self-government—the sort of thing which does sometimes happen in schools which claim to be " self-governing." I do not want to give the impression that the boys " did it all themselves," as I have often heard adults trying to do, and have wondered whether they were deceiving themselves or merely trying to deceive me ; on the other hand you will be very far amiss if you assume that it was a pretty normal kind of regime, with the boys " allowed to decide " certain things, so long as they decided in the way I wanted them to decide. During the first three months there was extreme disorder, and it must not be forgotten that we resolutely refused to inflict any kind of punishment or deal with any kind of difficult situation except by the method of an appeal to the community. The fact is, however, that the adults (and that meant in practice chiefly Kenneth and me) were automatically looked upon as the persons responsible for seeing that breaches of the law were brought before the community, and in many ways we accepted a good deal of responsibility that had not been formally given to us by the meeting. We got the boys up in the mornings, " supervised " their activities throughout the day, and put them to bed at night. The teacher conducted " his " school in his own way, and we had no official connection with that. After 18 months things had become pretty orderly and life was rather too much a matter of routine for my liking. I was wondering what I should do about this when Frankie Fox did it for me.

CHAPTER FIVE

RESPONSIBILITIES SHARED

" The Constitution bored him and he slew it."
G. K. CHESTERTON—" The Revolutionist : *or* Lines to a Statesman."

FRANKIE, and one or two of his cronies had, by reason of much trespassing, pilfering and other misdemeanours been " unfree men " for some time, and were suffering divers other disabilities, the result of the community's efforts to check their anti-social propensities. They began to despair of ever emerging from their present restricted state, and it was then that Frankie conceived his brilliant idea, which was to have such a tremendous effect on the life of Barns. He said, " Why don't we start Barns all over again ? " —but was unable at first to think of any good reason why we should. I was very happy to provide him with a few—as that we had now a large number of boys who had not enjoyed the experience of helping to build a system of government ; that the system we had was getting top-heavy with rules and regulations and restrictions and prohibitions . . . and so on. At the next meeting Frankie brought forward his idea, which all considered an excellent one. It was put to the meeting, carried *nemine contradicente*, and the Chairman proceeded to the next item on the agenda. It seemed to me, however, that before leaving this matter, some kind of arrangements should be made for the new start, or at least some preparations made for the interim period. Instead of saying so outright, however, I gave what was intended to be a little prompting. " Just a minute, Mr. Chairman," I said, " You've just decided to abolish the House meeting—ought we to be going on to the next item ? " There was a moment's pause while this was taken in. Then there was a loud whoop and all the boys rushed out of the room !

I confess that I was not prepared for this, and was a little doubtful what to do next. It seemed to me that the " old hands " should not have been so irresponsible as to leave us with no form of government, and no indication as to how one was to be brought into being. On the other hand, if we were literally to " start all over again" the presumption was that I should gradually introduce the boys to the idea of shared responsibility, as I had originally done. That seemed just too artificial. So after thinking it over I dropped a bombshell. After breakfast the next morning I said something to this effect : " Last night the House meeting was scrapped and it was decided that Barns should be started all over again. Well, when we first started there was only one boy, then six, a bit later eleven, and so on ; we grew gradually. As I am, according to many people, a bit of a fool, I allowed those boys to do pretty well what they liked. They had pretty nearly. absolute freedom, and that freedom was after a time limited by themselves when it was found that some people didn't know how to use it. We established as nearly as possible a democracy. But that isn't the usual way of starting places like this. They're usually a dictatorship. Freedom is limited to the very minimum, though the dictator may expand it a little as time goes on. Well—we're starting again, but don't assume —since you seem to be leaving everything to me—that I shall act now exactly as I did then. I've decided to act in the usual way, and set up a dictatorship. There are thirty boys here now, not a dozen, and to be perfectly frank, I'm not prepared to take the risk of pretending I don't know that some of those boys don't know how to use freedom. *They* might not mind getting into trouble with our neighbours, but as most people consider *me* responsible for *your* behaviour, I'm not prepared to run the risk of looking a bigger fool in the neighbourhood than I look already. When there were just a few new boys I could use the excuse that I didn't know they were like that—I haven't got that excuse now. So all right, we're starting again, and this time we're starting as a dictatorship. I'm the dictator, and you'll jolly well do as you're told, do it smartly, and no back-answers. There are no free men, and no-one goes outside Barns except with the official party—if and when there is one. *I* will dictate the orderly system, *I* will make all the rules, and if you don't like 'em you shouldn't have been in such a hurry to surrender your freedom when you had it.

Rule one is that any boy who isn't in the Dining Room by the time Grace has been said, is too late for that meal. Rule two is that when the bell rings for school you will all assemble in the hall to be counted, and not just drift into school when you feel like it. I'll announce the next rules as we go along. We're going to have a bit of discipline in this place for a change. In your own interests I advise you to take this very seriously. If you think you can ignore *my* rules like some of you did the rules of the House meeting, you'll be in for a nasty jolt." By this time there was an uneasy silence in the room. It all sounded very unpleasant (as I meant it to !), and people must have been wondering whatever had come over me. But I had not finished. " There will be one important difference between me and other dictators," I said. "As a rule you can only get rid of a dictator by bumping him off. I am going to be one of the rare exceptions. Any time you like to establish some kind of democratic assembly that wants to take over the job of running the house, I'll stand down. But it must be the real thing, not just a sham like the House meeting, whose rules were honoured more in the breach than in the observance, which did everything the adults suggested, and which anyway left most of the work to Ben and me" (For Ben was with us now ; I was being very hard on the House meeting—much harder than the circumstances warranted ; but like a good actor I exaggerated a little in order to get my point across). "I shall be ready and willing to hand over to anybody that will *really* run the place, from getting up to bedtime, seven days a week." Then I announced the orderly rota, and dismissed them from the Dining Room, one table at a time.

I kept it up, and incidentally I was astonished to find how amenable they were to discipline. Whyever any one should need a strap I cannot imagine. They "tried it on," of course, to see whether I was in earnest, and I believe it was really useful for them to discover that my previous lack of discipline had been because I would not, and not because I could not. Nevertheless, there was no punishment to speak of. Several boys went without breakfast one day because they weren't there in time, but that didn't happen again ; and I believe I did send a boy to bed one evening for something or other, but by and large, the infliction of discipline on these "difficult" boys was what is sometimes known as a "cinch."

But I didn't have to keep it up for long. After a week had elapsed a meeting was called of "all those who want to end the dictatorship." About half the boys attended the meeting, and as I had made it clear that I should be glad to help in any way, I was invited and attended. Wally Straight (aged 12) was elected to the Chair, and opened the meeting with a few well-chosen words, of which the following is the official record : "The Chairman (Wally Straight) told the meeting that they now had an opportunity to organise Barns all over again, and to do things the way they wanted them done. He said that it was up to the meeting to prove that Barns' boys could look after themselves." (Oddly enough there is no record of who was appointed Secretary, and was therefore responsible for the admirable minutes, but I think it was Ted Bounce).

Then I butted in and asked if I might say a few words. On permission being given, I reminded them that I was only going to surrender my authority to a properly constituted body that would really do the job, and explained what " the job " was. Then I said that one of the weaknesses of the House meeting had been that it was overweighted with adults so that some boys were reluctant to speak their minds. I didn't want the new thing to have the same disability, so I proposed to step outside, but if they wanted advice on any specific point they could call me in. Then I withdrew, though I have to confess that (as the meeting was in the Dining Room) I did a little eavesdropping through the lift hatch.

It was an extremely rowdy meeting and several boys were ejected for failing to respect the Chair. I was called in for advice on two or three points, withdrawing each time after I had said my piece.

Two or three meetings were necessary before everything was cleared up, and what came to birth was " The Citizens' Association." The name, I am sorry to say, was mine—they couldn't think of one themselves—but the constitution they evolved was entirely theirs.

The Citizens' Association might be described, in brief, as an oligarchy of the Elect. Membership was open to anyone who could " prove that he was willing to work for Barns." We were all frightfully excited and pleased about the new developments. I wrote several long letters to our Chairman, keeping her posted with the latest events. Reading them through to refresh my memory recalls very vividly the spirit and atmosphere of the time, and I think I cannot do better than quote from them. " . . . It was undoubtedly the most serious and purposeful meeting we have had here. The Citizens' Association took over forthwith. They put themselves to bed and supervised themselves in the bathroom. The following morning, Tuesday, my day off, sometimes known as " racket day," they got themselves up and did all that was necessary with no adult supervision at all, and May says the dormitories were cleaner than she has ever known them. The Chairman of the Citizens' Association took charge of the Dining Room, ringing the bell for Grace, and so on. And so they continued until bedtime, when they put themselves to bed. Everything did not go smoothly, by any means. There were various contingencies for which they had not legislated in advance ; there were conflicting interpretations of such rules as had been made ; some boys were jealous of those in office—and so on. But from all accounts it seems to have been as well-ordered and peaceful a Tuesday as we have had for some time. But there was one very interesting piece of back-wash. They were so rebellious in school that teacher had the greatest difficulty in getting any order at all, and spent the whole of the first period haranguing them ! Stuart Wild " ran away " (publicly, with a broad grin on his face) and teacher . . . fetched him back again—*and asked Ben to deal with him !* Ben took him into his room, where he did as good a morning's work as he has ever done. Ben and I have left them very much to themselves when they have been carrying out their new functions of " looking after themselves " in the morning and evening, because we wanted to impress upon them the fact that they *are* looking after themselves.   But after a day or two we shall insinuate ourselves again, but in a different relationship—we shall be more " one of the boys " instead of the person in authority.   It is going to be very difficult to keep going, but very fruitful, I think."

The " little bit of back-wash" developed in time into something more like a tidal wave, but that belongs to another chapter.* I wrote Mary Smith again a few days later . . . " I'm glad you are as thrilled as I am about the " Citizens." They have been going nearly a week now, which is quite a long time in the life of an eleven-year-old, and things are still going well.   If they keep it up for two weeks, I shall begin to feel that it is going to last.   I find it very difficult to prevent myself getting fearfully excited about it.   Yesterday, I thought I would like to go and meet Ruth (who had been away), arriving Edinburgh early in the afternoon, and after much pondering I decided to take the afternoon off and go. I would never have thought of going during the old regime, but I thought it might increase their confidence in themselves and also serve as a kind of a test just to see how they could manage.   Of course Ben was there, but the second in command never has had a great deal of authority,† and it has always been customary to have two men on duty all the time at week-ends.   Well—everything seems to have gone very well except that one boy—Jack McKay— was very difficult.   But that doesn't mean anything.   He is in the stage that Stuart Wild was in a year ago.   He has been, on my suggestion, removed from the jurisdiction of the Citizens' Association, because " people can only look after themselves, and join in with other people, if they are happy, and anyone can see that he isn't." Some of the Citizens—especially the Chairman—remember the time when *they* were not so happy, so they understand what I am talking about.   So he was put in my special charge, and they call him now my " patient " ; their idea, not mine.   I should never think of calling a boy a patient, not at any rate in conversation with him."

* See page 101.

† Or hadn't had up to then—that was before Ben had established himself ; and anyway, after the formation of the C.A. the personal authority of adults was of far less significance than hitherto.

Membership of the Citizens' Association consisted at first of those who had attended the first meeting and had expressed their willingness to " help Barns "—there were thirteen of them. Thereafter, new members had to be nominated by a Citizen and approved by a majority of the Association. Every Citizen had to take his turn as " Officer on Duty," two being appointed for each day. The Officers on Duty were, in short, responsible for the orderly carrying out of the routine from rising in the morning until " Lights Out " at night. It was quickly recognised that the Officers on Duty were not exercising a personal authority, but were acting on behalf of the community as a whole, and we were amused as well as pleased to see that one of the smallest boys (wee Sandy Sporran) seemed to exercise greater authority than the biggest boy in the place—Alf Blake. The Citizens (rather to my alarm) declared that all members of the Association—and no others—were " Freemen." I was more nervous about this than subsequent events justified, for anyone who behaved in an unsuitable manner—*i.e.*, who acted as a hindrance instead of a help to Barns—was quickly relieved of his membership and had to " prove himself" before being re-admitted. The Officers of the Association formed a Committee to hear charges, meeting each day. As no adult was an officer, the Committee met without any adult being present—unless he were present as plaintiff or defendant ; or unless he were a spectator. Though it should be added that I was sometimes present as " Counsel for the Defence."

There was a time when I thought the whole thing was going to " flop." Wally Straight, after a few weeks, found the responsibility too much for him and resigned the Chairmanship, and Jacob Everson was appointed in his place. Jacob, though 13 years of age, was very childish and irresponsible. I used to worry about him a good deal because we didn't seem to touch him at all. He seemed to be entirely spineless, and drifted this way and that with every idle wind that blew. I did not conceal my disgust at this appointment. I said we all liked Jacob, and he was a charming boy ; but that was not a sufficient reason for making him Chairman. I was making a fool of myself. The boys seemed to understand Jacob's character better than I. For three or four months he was an ideal Chairman—sensitive to the feelings of the meeting, resolute and conscientious in seeing that those decisions were implemented. I was astonished and delighted, and had the pleasure of confessing to Jacob how much I had misjudged him. I remember vividly a scene I happened upon outside the dormitories one evening. Jacob, tears streaming from his eyes and blood from his nose, was hanging on to the bully of the place, Martin Dodd, who had been ordered to bed until he was prepared to do his orderly duty. He had refused to go to bed and the Chairman, disdaining help from anyone, started *putting* him to bed ! He succeeded, too. It was, of course, a tactical error to attempt the use of physical violence at all (as I explained to Jacob afterwards), but the pluck and fortitude displayed were admirable, and I was never again able to think of him as spineless.

The Citizens' Association lasted about eight months. Its end (a dissolution by common consent) was brought about by a variety of factors which for several reasons I cannot here describe. But I was quite glad to see it end because, though an admirable institution, and one which was a turning point in the history of Barns, I was afraid that it was giving perhaps more responsibility to some boys than they were old enough to bear. It was a suitable and necessary re-action to the House meeting, but I thought the time was approaching when the happy mean might be sought. In any case, I am not in favour of one system going on too long, because I think there is, if anything, more value in devising and initiating a system of living together than there is in working it, though of course, it must also be worked.

Well—we have had several systems since then, some good, some bad and some indifferent, but I will not burden the reader by describing them all in full. Sometimes they were devised by the boys, more often they arose out of suggestions I made, though my suggestions were often improved upon. We have never had anything that was so completely the work of the boys as the Citizens' Association. At present we enjoy government by a cabinet which is answerable to the " General Meeting," meeting weekly. General meeting once consisted of everyone, now it is limited to freemen, though others may attend, and, I believe, they are allowed to express an opinion, but not to vote. The Prime Minister recently decided to call himself the President, but his functions remain the same, namely to keep his ministers in order ! There is a Minister in charge of each department of the life of the place. At one time there was a Minister of Occupations, a Minister of Routine, a Minister of Work, a Minister of School, a Minister of Justice (the Cabinet, rather oddly, acting as a Court !) and a Minister of Money. Recently there has been something of a re-organisation because each Dormitory has been asked to elect a " gang-leader " (the gang-leaders acting as a Court under the Chairmanship of the " President ") and the number of Ministers has been reduced. We are all taxed—adults and Ministers paying double what everyone else pays—it is usually a halfpenny or a penny a week, according to the state of the exchequer—and one of its principal uses is the payment of " salaries " to the Ministers ! The Chairman of the General Meeting presides in the Dining Room at meal times and his word is law—not because he's Bobby Dodd (though naturally, there are good Chairmen and bad Chairmen) but because he's the Chairman. When I compare the orderly state of the Dining Room at meal times now—whether there's an adult present or not—compared with what it used to be at one time with all the adults present ; and reflect that all this has been brought about by our refusing to accept authority and pushing it onto the boys, I am in no doubt about the value of " shared responsibility ! "

To all of this there is a curious kind of ambivalence in the attitude of the boys. They appreciate " having their freedom," they enjoy and yet I believe they would surrender their share of " shared responsibility " any day with pleasure. Ruth and I went to visit another children's hostel, and told the boys where we were going. When we got back, Frankie Fox said to Ruth, " Do they have their freedom there like we do here ? " Ruth had to tell him that they did not. " I bet Mr. Wills and Kenney would soon change that if they were there," he said. (That was in the early days before I had attained the dignity of " Willsy.") So they do appreciate " their freedom," and they do unquestionably learn that the price of freedom is eternal vigilance—*and* a lot of hard work. Sometimes we have wondered whether the whole thing was not going to collapse, because of the reluctance of boys to take office. At first a boy will be delighted with the idea of being an official of some kind—no doubt it is associated in his mind with the idea of being a Monitor and getting privileges of various kinds from the teacher. He soon finds out his mistake, for Privilege has not yet found its way into our Democracy, except for the privileges (or some of them) associated with adulthood. He enjoys for a time being in the public eye, and the feeling of being someone of importance. Then he finds he has to give up a game to do part of his job, or he has to do something which may make him unpopular. Then, if he is conscientious, he makes the required sacrifice—or he resigns ; if not, he finds himself after a day or two being " sacked." When that has happened a few times the Meeting is reduced to appointing nonentities, because no-one else will have the jobs. Sometimes the nonentity proves to have been not such a nonentity after all—as in the case of Jacob Everson. But more often he is just a " flop," and things go from bad to worse. Then interest in " shared responsibility " reaches a very low ebb, indeed, and none of the boys seem to mind very much. I imagine the reason they do not mind is that they know that if the worst comes to the worst and the adults were to seize the reigns of government, there would be nothing to worry about. In spite of my assumed ferocity the week before the Citizens' Association was formed, they know that neither I nor my colleagues are really ferocious, and that our regime would be mild and beneficent—as well as efficient! So why, they feel (I do not say it is conscious ratiocination)—why should we have all the bother and worry of running things when the presumed alternative is so little to be feared?

We are not the first democracy to have experienced this difficulty. Did not the great Augustus resort eventually to the expedient of inflicting heavy fines upon the Senators who neglected their duties? An apt analogy, the cynic will say. That wily old bird went out of his way to delude the Romans into the belief that they were a democracy of sorts, while taking great pains to see to it that the effective control was in his own hands. They, on the other hand, so far as they saw through his little game, saw that his administration was a better one than they had enjoyed for some time, and were prepared to leave things to him. But it isn't exactly like that with us because our citizens are, after all, children, not responsible adults, and a certain measure of authority must remain in the hands of the adults if the children are not to be unhealthy or unhappy.

We can very often see such a period of slackness approaching, and in such a case our policy is a well-defined one. When things are going well, we help the various officers as much as they need help, though without actually relieving them of any responsibility, and sometimes take steps to see that any little lapses do not have too serious consequences. During a " slack " period, however, we remove our supporting hand and allow things to take their course. In the normal course of events, I should not mind reminding an otherwise competent " Minister of Money," if he was very busy with a game on Saturday morning, that he has to see about the paying of the "salaries" of his fellow ministers. During a slack period, however, I should forget it, too—after all, it's no business of mine !—and there would be the ministers with no salaries. I am even guilty too, I fear, of playing what might seem like dirty little tricks. Normally, if the Officer on Duty forgets to put the games away, I might point out this omission to the appropriate minister. But I have been known during a slack period to " steal " the billiard balls. This may seem a little hard, but in fact it is better for the balls to be " stolen " by me (from whom they are recoverable) than for them to be taken outside by some irresponsible boy and dropped in the Tweed. This is, of course, especially the case in wartime, when such things are practically irreplaceable. After a week or two, things get pretty chaotic—and then one of the more responsible boys accepts office, and there is a fresh start— perhaps with an entirely different system.

This is not a text-book on how to run an institution for " difficult " children on self-governing lines, because so much depends on the personalities of the people concerned and the kind of relationship that exists between them, that it is impossible for one person to lay down a set of rules for another to follow. At the same time I am only writing this in the hope that it will encourage others to attempt the same *sort* of thing, and to those I should like to utter a few words of advice.

The first is that " shared responsibility " is no picnic for the adults. Workers in more orthodox establishments visiting Barns and finding our boys, for example, quietly putting themselves to bed (yes, even quietly, sometimes !) might think " How pleasant for the staff not to have dormitory duties at night " and if they were very superficial people they might find several such pleasant things in the life of Barns. Such persons are advised never to attempt any kind of experimenting in this field. " Shared responsibility " (though no evil spirit) cometh not forth but by prayer and fasting, and any concerned in it will find not merely a touch at the hem of their garment, but a constant clinging thereto, and will find that much virtue goes out of them daily.

The next point is that it is utterly futile to attempt to make use of this method unless you have complete faith in its value. In no circumstances must it be tried " to see if it works." In those circumstances it doesn't.

Thirdly—so far as the children or the democratic assembly are given authority, that authority must be absolute. I have said this before, but it is worth repeating. It is better to limit the sphere of the children's responsibility to something very small, if that authority is absolute, than to give them a wide but vague sphere of control with the danger that you might step in one day and veto a decision that they have made. ' But you will find, if you have confidence in them, that you are repeatedly being astonished by their wisdom.

Do not look for efficiency. If you want that you must provide it in the good old way. This is learning by doing in a very real sense, and nothing is learnt if no mistakes are made.

Finally—and this is the most important point of all—shared responsibility is not the first plank in our platform, and it should

not be the first plank in anyone else's.   Because it obtrudes itself
somewhat, and introduces features that are a novelty to many people,
some think it is the most important thing about our method.   That
is very far from the case.   We use it for reasons which I hope are
by now clear to the reader, even if they have not all been explicitly
stated.   But it is merely a corollary to our primary instrument—
the instrument of love.   First, foremost, and all the time the children
must feel themselves to be loved.   Most of us have grown up in
families where authority was wielded by someone of whose love we
were confident.   Many of these children have had a different
experience, and they are apt to be unable to reconcile love and
authority.   So we try to separate them a little.   Their fellow
inmates wield authority on behalf of the community (not on
behalf of the adults, like a Prefect or any other kind of quisling),
and it is gradually learnt that love and authority are not necessarily
mutually exclusive.   At the same time our own contact is not
marred from the start by our having an authoritarian attitude
and the child thus more easily believes himself loved.   But
the *primary* thing is the love—seek ye first the kingdom of heaven
and its righteousness, and all these things shall be added unto you.

CHAPTER SIX

COUNSELS OF PERFECTION

"Come, my songs, let us speak of perfection—
We shall get ourselves rather disliked."
EZRA POUND—" Personæ."

I WAS having a private talk with Jimmy Gay. " I've been giving you a rough time lately, haven't I ? " I had, too. I had had a feeling that it wouldn't do Jimmy any harm to be told just how his behaviour was liable to strike people. I do not know exactly why I felt the time to be ripe for this. A large proportion of one's work in what Aichorn calls " The therapy of the dis-social " is intuitive. Heavy tomes may be (and are !) written about why one should do this and when one should do that ; but any work which ignores the value of intuition is ignoring a great deal—I should say about half the subject. Not that one can write much about intuitive judgments. One makes them and one acts on them, and that's about all there is to it.* Their value increases with one's experience, and I very much doubt whether anyone will have a great deal of success in this work whose intuitive judgments are not sound.

James, then, was inclined to be a bully, he was extremely thought-less of other people's convenience and comfort, he dodged his orderly duties whenever he could, and in general was a pest, and a complete liability in the body politic. Feeling then, as I say, intuitively, that this would be the right medicine just now, I had been giving him " what for." Any time I found he had committed any small delinquency I gave him a good " row," called him many hard names, and in general made myself thoroughly objectionable to him. When I thought things had gone far enough ; when, that is, I began to think Jimmy was looking at me in a kind of way in which I don't like to be looked at, I sought an opportunity for a private talk with him.

He agreed that I had been giving him a rough time—" Aye, ye have that " . . . " I've called you a lot of nasty names, haven't I ? " . . . " Aye, ye have that " . . . " I can't like you very

* I am not attaching any mystical or esoteric significance to intuition, at which I scoffed a good deal when I was younger. By it I simply mean decisions based on experience which is not recalled to consciousness at the time of the decision, but which is, nevertheless, present in the pre-conscious or the unconscious.

much if I call you all those names, can I ? " . . . " Aye, ye can."
. . . " Oh, what makes you think that ? " . . . " Geikie tellt
me " . . . " Geikie told you ? What on earth do you mean ?
What's *he* been saying to you ?·" " He tellt me that if Willsy calls
you a lot of names an' that, he still likes ye."

So I confirmed the mental tick I had long since placed against
Jimmy's name, but which I had been afraid recent circumstances
might have blurred somewhat. He still knew that I loved him.

That is the first, the fundamental, the absolutely essential pre-
requisite of the " therapy of the dis-social." They must feel that they
are loved.

" Love," said Augustine of Hippo, " and do what you will."
Like all such aphoristic generalisations, this one must not be taken
too literally, but if I were forbidden to write a book and compelled
instead to write a sentence, that would be the sentence. The system
under which we are all brought up has many faults. I, myself, have
said many hard things about parents, and hope I may be spared to
say many more. But this is one of those cases where the shadow
proves the light. The fact that there is a number of unsatisfactory
parents and unsatisfactory homes serves to remind us how very
satisfactory the generality of homes and parents are. A girl gets
married at any age between 17 and 30 and starts breeding children.
She may be almost illiterate, she will probably have no theoretical
knowledge whatever of rearing children, and no practical
knowledge except such as comes from watching and sometimes
helping her mother—who, again, started out equally ill-equipped.
Yet, by and large, they make a pretty good job of it. Why ? How ?
Whence comes this skill ? The answer is—and I must run the risk
of appearing unforgivably sentimental—love. The girl loves her
offspring, and all the rest seems to follow. She makes mistakes—
sometimes stupid mistakes—but more often than not she seems to
rectify them, and although there are neurotics and delinquents and
invalids in the world, most of us are a credit to what must seem, on
any rational grounds, a very slipshod, hit-or-miss sort of method.
Love and common-sense seem to be the principal requisites, and if a
girl has these, the chances are that she won't go far wrong. I am
always a little nervous when I see young mothers going all
psychological. They don't need it, and the chances are they will
start practising some high-falutin, half-understood idea in defiance
of their own intuitive judgments, to the great detriment of the child.
I was once so ill-advised, when I was a good deal younger than I
am now, as to deliver a lecture to an assembly of working-class
mothers, on the bringing-up of children. It seemed to me an

excellent lecture, full of progressive ideas, which would be very good for the mothers and children concerned. When the Chairman asked if there were any questions or comments, a voice from the back of the hall was heard to say, in loud clear tones—" Yes. Wait till you've had half-a-dozen of your own, then call another meeting." Well—I don't know that she wasn't right. They knew they didn't need all that stuff—they were doing on the whole a pretty satisfactory job without it, with their native wit and their affection.

The young baby clings in a physical sense to its mother, who, by supporting it and feeding it, gives it physical security and physical strength. In like manner by loving it, and being loved by it, she provides it with emotional strength and security. And the same goes for the father. He also loves his progeny, unless there is something wrong with him, and although it may be less obvious, he has as important a part to play as the mother. He also by loving the child helps to create that sheet anchor for the emotions, and like her, all he has to do is to be himself—his natural self— and if he is any good at all, all will be well. Though it must be added that, paradoxically, they both provide a measure of security also by their prohibitions and compulsions, as well as by their more obvious manifestations of affection.

The main ingredients then, of a successful home (apart from the physical necessities and conveniences) are a mother, a father, love and common-sense. And the greatest of these is love. When one of the ingredients is missing, the offspring may find their way into hospitals, child guidances clinics, courts, approved schools or— into Barns. For we have seen, in chapter three, what kind of homes Barns boys tend to come from. Three-quarters of them are *known* to be families where one or more of the ingredients are missing, and only two boys out of fifty are positively known to come from a family which apparently has all the ingredients—though I made no effort in chapter three to assess the ingredient I have referred to here as common-sense. Apart from common-sense, the absence of any one ingredient means also the absence of love. How can a boy be loved by his father if he has no father ? How can a boy feel himself to be loved by his mother if his mother has deserted and gone to live with another man ? For love, in this case, is like justice in the well-known maxim to the effect that it is not enough for justice to have been done ; justice must manifestly appear to have been done. It is not enough for a child to be loved ; the child must know himself to be loved. That is why I sometimes say that if a child seems almost unloveable, at least we can try to go through the motions. It is better to create a false impression that a child is loved (though I doubt whether that can ever be done successfully) than to create a false impression that he is not. A good deal of the trouble with our Fox brothers was due to this very thing. They were not certain of their mother's affection. She came to see them one visiting day, and when she was ready to go I collected them up and said rather fatuously, "Come along and kiss your mother goodbye." She laughed. "They won't do that," she said. "What, won't kiss their mother?" . . . "Oh no, Mr. Fox and me haven't brought them up to be like that. We don't want them to be sloppy." When they went home for a holiday at Christmas, they were simply weighed down with presents they had acquired for their parents—trying, as it seemed to me, to buy a little affection. She was fond of them really, but the ingredient of common-sense was lacking.

If, then, so many of the children who come to us have been deprived of this fundamental necessity, manifestly we must provide it. That is our first job, it is our most important job, and it is our most difficult job. For when I speak of love I do mean love—I do mean the kind of feeling a parent has for his children. I do not mean the esteem which a child can earn from the adults in its environment by being " a good boy." I do not mean the benign and somewhat affectionate feeling that a teacher might feel for his class when everything is going steadily forward. The kind of thing I am thinking of has no relation to the behaviour of the child, and is not influenced by it. It cannot be bought with goodness nor lost by misbehaviour. However often she may say it, a mother never means, " You've been a very naughty boy and mother doesn't love you any more." And neither must we. Indeed, we must never say it. A mother who is confident of her relationship may risk such a remark, but we may not. *George Sand, it seems to me, sums up the matter admirably :—

" Make children feel that they are loved, but make them understand, too, that the love of parents is very different from that of friends. Convince them that parental affection will always be there waiting for them, whatever their faults, because the tender affection of parents withstands every test. But make them recognise that the affection of friends is the result of esteem, confidence and choice. Children must learn that friendship is based on merit, and that it is won or lost according as they are strong or weak, devoted to others or egotistically centred on self." The kind of affection we—the adults—at Barns try to shew is the first kind, the parental affection. The other kind may or may not be earned from the community at

* " Intimate Journal," translated by Marie Jenney Howe, page 73.

large or from other individuals in it. That is why we have our machinery of Shared Responsibility. The concern of the adults is with the unconscious emotional life of the child—to provide a sheet anchor for the emotions, to establish that security which the home has (so often) failed to provide. Shared Responsibility— the meetings, the Courts, the committees—provide a vehicle for the expression of public opinion, and it is through this that the child learns—this time through conscious cerebration, and through experience—how to earn the esteem and affection of ordinary acquaintances. But of that I have already spoken. At present I am concerned with the establishment of security through affection, and the task of the adults.

It is not just a matter of being " awfully fond of children." Anyone can be that. It is a matter of being " awfully fond " of Johnny Jones whose table manners are nauseating (he sits opposite you and crams as much food into his mouth as he possibly can ; this he chews with his big mouth wide open ; presently he lets out a loud guffaw, ejecting his breath powerfully through his overful and open mouth . . .) ; it is a matter of being " awfully fond " of Willie Smith whose nose is usually in a condition such as to make one retch almost every time one sees it ; it is a matter of being " awfully fond " of Jimmy Brown, who stinks because of his encopresis ; or even of Tommy Green, who has all these failings and a foul and nasty disposition thrown in. In consists of loving this Tommy Green in spite of all that, of making him feel that this affection is always there, is something on which he can absolutely rely, which will never fail, whatever he may do. It consists of establishing a relationship such that, however much the child may wound his own self-esteem, he cannot damage the esteem in which we hold him. The sort of relationship we want to set up is the very happy relationship which seemed to exist between David Scrivens and his father. David had no mother, and his father had just joined the Navy. The day he heard that his father had joined the Navy, Kenneth Roberton happened to be just behind him at a time when he thought he was alone. He was talking to himself. He was saying " My Daddy, my Daddy. He's in the Navy now. My Daddy's in the Navy. But he's still my Daddy. He's still my Daddy, although he's in the Navy. *He can't break out of me.*" When that relationship is established, therapy has begun.

That, then, is the task we set ourselves. God knows we fail often enough. But however often we miss the mark, and however widely, that is the aim. One of the results is that a boy always

E

seems to get worse when he comes to Barns because, being anxious not to mar the establishment of that relationship at the outset, we tend to ignore his social failings. We may even, on occasion, approve them. If a boy's only claim to distinction is his history of anti-social activity, then we help him to establish himself with us by lending an appreciative ear to his account of his depredations. We'll give him something better to boast about later on ; in the meantime that's all he's got, and it's a jolly sight more than some people have, and more worthy of praise very often than a whole lifetime of negative obscurity. In the same way we often appear to be encouraging bad language, because one of the worst barriers between street boys and respectable adults is that the need to watch one's tongue causes restraint. For these are not your middle-class children to whom swearing is a delicious novelty and who have a phase and grow out of it. It is their native idiom, and one has to understand it. Your respectable adult, who is shocked by bad language, never enjoys the experience of being called, with a mixture of admiration and affection, " You bloody old sod." It is often pure love when I am called " You bald-headed old bugger." But even when it is what we all understand it to be, we don't think it important enough to risk messing things up at the start, so that we once heard a boy boasting, after he had been here a week or two, " I can swear in front of Benjy now ! " God bless him. I haven't heard him swear for weeks.

Obviously, a certain amount of discretion has to be used. We cannot allow a new boy always to do exactly everything he wants to do, and he would not like it if we did. That in itself would be a form of neglect which might mean that we didn't care for him. Here, again, one has to rely largely upon intuition, but of course we have at Barns a machinery of government which works more or less independently of adults and prevents serious breaches of routine and good order. Certainly when the relationship has once been established it is possible to be remarkably frank and outspoken about a boy's failings because he realises that one *is* talking about his failings, and not about *him*. That is why—to return to where I started—I was pleased to find that Jimmy Gay had not been put off by what I had been saying to him—he knew I still loved him.

CHAPTER SEVEN

PSYCHOLOGICAL FIRST-AID

" The young Scout must be taught that the object of first-aid is not to make him a sort of amateur doctor, but only to prevent harm being done until expert attention can be given, and to attend to anything that requires immediate attention . . . "
"Boy Scout Tests and How to Pass Them."

I HAVE known occasions indeed when I have had a most fierce and violent row with a boy so that I was spluttering with rage and he in tears. A quarter of an hour later we have met in my private room for a weekly talk and have chatted amicably together with absolutely no reference to—and no thought of—the squabble we had just had.

It seems to me that in these circumstances there is set up something very much akin to what Psycho-analysts call " the analytical situation." Whatever else this may mean (and I do not profess to understand it very fully) it clearly involves certain important elements arising out of the relationship between the analyst and the patient. In the first place there is the transference—that is to say, the direction to the analyst of some measure of the feelings originally directed to the first love-object—the parents. This has aspects both of love and hate, but the " positive," or love aspects, will usually predominate in a successful analysis. In the second place the patient recognises in the analyst not a person who is there to lay down the moral laws or to enumerate educational principles. Questions of " good " and " bad " and " ought " do not come to the forefront of discussions. The analyst is recognised as a person who will never fail to appreciate the point of view of the patient, and who is out for the same end as the patient. In these circumstances, and only in these circumstances, the analyst carries on his work, though doubtless the analytical situation involves more than just that. But I find that it is in these circumstances, too, that I am best able to carry on my own work. It is widely held and proclaimed by writers of the psychoanalytic school that it is not possible for anyone in the relationship of teacher, parent, or similar person to establish this relationship, because they are necessarily concerned with prohibitions and compulsions and the insistence on a point of view which the child sees as at variance with his own. I do not find it impossible. I find that it is possible for me to take up, and for the children to recognise in me a dual rôle. On the one hand I am the Warden—the person ultimately responsible for the good conduct of the House and all in it—however much I may by delegation share that responsibility. On the other hand I am Willsy, to whom one can talk with the utmost freedom about anything and who can always appreciate one's point of view. The degree to which the boys are able to distinguish between these two functions often astonishes me, and I would not at one time have thought it possible. Upon examination, however, it is perhaps not as improbable as it may seem, and may indeed serve a very useful purpose by splitting up the ambivalence—the negative side is directed to the Warden, with his restrictions and prohibitions, the positive to Wills. There is thus far less of the conflict and confusion which may arise from having both these kinds of feeling towards the same person.

I am not trying to suggest that everyone at Barns clearly distinguishes between my two functions ; but a fair portion distinguish clearly, and another fair portion less clearly. But in case of doubt I can usually establish the " Willsy " relationship by taking a boy into my private room. This room is not my sitting room, nor is it my office :* I use it only for talking to boys in my "Willsy" capacity. We do not discuss any present troubles the boy may be going through unless he raises them, and then my attitude is very carefully a non-moral one, viewing the thing purely from the boy's point of view rather from the point of view of authority or society—though I may sometimes add, if it seems expedient, a word about how some other people might view the matter.

These interviews may take place sporadically because the occasion seems to demand it ; but they also take place at regular intervals. Normally I see every boy in turn at the rate of two a night on the night I am free from routine duties—that is· to say, about six or eight boys a week. The first will come along at 8 o'clock, is given a sweet (rationing notwithstanding) and told that he will have to go at 8.10 promptly by the clock on the table. At 8.10 he goes and the second boy comes at 8.15, leaving at 8.25. A boy feels much more at his ease if he knows exactly how long he is going to stay. How many of us who are older and wiser have never mastered the technique of getting up and going ! I make the interview end at the appointed time even if we are in the middle of an interesting conversation—we can always, if necessary, continue it to-morrow night ! Another important point about these discussions is that

---

* I seem to have an enormous suite of rooms. In theory the room in question s the spare bedroom ; my office is the staff common-room.

they are not only strictly confidential, but they are never (so far as I can manage it !) carried over into my other relationship. Jimmy Gay is an interesting example of this, too. He is a great raconteur and can be seen at almost any time holding a group of boys spellbound with his stories. We were talking about his stories in my room one day, and I said what a good idea it would be to write some of them down. He thought it would be a good idea too, so I bought him an imposing-looking manuscript book to write them down in, and every now and then he comes and reads them to me. Another time we were talking about his own adventures—which have been not a few, chiefly taking long journeys on the backs of lorries and getting himself sent home by the Police by rail. I mentioned in a casual sort of way that he always seemed to be truanting in those days, but not now. " Ah, weel, ye ken," he said, " Schule's guid here."

To-day I was presiding at the Committee (I am President this month. This is very unusual, but we won't go into that now) and Jimmy was brought before us by the Officer on Duty, on a charge of being late for school, of mucking up a lesson, and of generally making himself a nuisance in school. Jimmy has had several such charges lately and indeed the General Meeting had to ask the Chairman to give him a talking-to about it. So we were pretty severe with Jimmy to-day. I gave him a real good row, referring to the way he made himself and other boys late by holding them in holes and corners with his stupid stories that no one but a chump would waste his time on. We weren't choosing our words with care, we were just fed up with Jimmy and—for the moment—with everything about him. The fact that at another time and in another place I myself had been very appreciative of the same " stupid " stories was neither here nor there. Jimmy didn't refer to it because I suppose he felt it belonged somewhere else, and because he vaguely realised that we were not to be taken exactly literally —the main thing was that he should understand how fed up with him his behaviour made us feel. But I was very careful not to say—" You're the twerp who said to me the other day that you don't truant now because school's good here, yet you make yourself a nuisance there and do your best to make it *bad*." If I had, he would have been very careful what he said to me in future.

Although I have ventured to make a comparison between my relation to the child, and that of a psychoanalyst, I should not for one moment like it to be thought that I regard myself as a psychoanalyst, or as any other kind of psychotherapist. I deprecate most strongly any attempt by laymen* to tinker about with a child's mind and my experience has been that those who know least about it are the most confident in setting themselves up as amateur psychotherapists. I have compared elsewhere† my position to that of the Matron of a hospital, whose function it is to provide the atmosphere in which the doctors can carry on their work, and to carry out the treatment prescribed by the doctors. In very many routine cases the nursing staff carry out the therapy from beginning to end, the medical staff merely watching to see that all is going according to plan. So, too, can the trained psychiatric social worker effect a certain amount of routine therapy by carrying out certain rules, keeping his eyes open, and using his common-sense.

The first function of these "therapeutic talks" (as I confess I call them privately, but of course not to the child) is that they are a means of taking special notice of the child—a thing which is always appreciated and which helps to create and maintain the feeling of being at least cared for. If they did nothing else they would justify themselves in that way. But one can also apply a certain amount of psychological first-aid. I have given a small example *en passant*—how, in conversation with Jimmy Gay, who only seemed to be able to get a sense of achievement through rebelliousness—I referred to his skill as a story teller and to the fact that he was no longer a truant. His stories I praised because I know he likes to regard them as an achievement. The cessation of truanting I merely drew his attention to casually, in case he had not noticed it, but here I neither praised nor blamed. No blame, because after all it is not blameworthy, and no praise because that might have associated me in his mind with the various authorities against whom, as a truant, he fought. But it may have implanted a little seed of pride which, if it grows, may lessen the need to seek a sense of achievement in other less desirable ways. Equally, of course, it may not, but at any rate no harm is done and there are many opportunities of dropping such seeds.

Arthur Collins is an example of something a little more positive than the mere dropping of a seed. Arthur was said to have a drunken and unfaithful father, an overbearing and ambitious mother who had no insight into his problems, and to have thought he was not wanted at home. We compared families—how many brothers and sisters we had, what our respective positions were in our families,

---

* By a layman I mean an untrained person, not merely a non-medical person. There are of course other kinds of psychological training besides the medical.

† " The Hawkspur Experiment"—George Allen & Unwin Ltd., 1941.

what our mothers and fathers were like. In spite of reports we had received about the father, Arthur seemed to have a genuinely warm feeling towards him, but there was marked reserve about his mother. Apropos nothing in particular, I told him of a funny episode in my own childhood. I was teasing my mother once when she was preparing some fish for cooking. She threatened in fun to lay about me with the fish unless I desisted. I dared her to do so, and we had a mock battle in which my mother chased me with a herring.*

" *My* mother," said Arthur, "chases me with a poker ! " " That's a more risky kind of joke than my mother's," I said. With a good deal of feeling Arthur replied, " It's no' a joke." No, it appeared that Mrs. Collins was quite serious in threatening him with a poker. It makes no difference if (as is quite possible) he had invented the whole thing. That is the sort of woman he conceived his mother to be. He described various episodes with vividness and feeling. "I bet you'd like to bend her over and lay about *her* with a poker," I said. He certainly would. There was no doubt about that, and from his description of how he would set about it, it was clear that that idea had not originated with *me*. He had obviously given the matter much thought, and considered himself very wicked for harbouring such ideas, which we may assume he had never expressed to anyone before. By sharing his phantasies with me he was able in some measure to " get them off his chest," and my unshocked attitude would lessen his feeling of guilt and shame. All this, of course, is just scratching on the surface, and I have no doubt that Arthur's desire to flog his mother's posterior had much more to it than a simple desire to get his own back. But that is something I cannot touch—it would need the services of a psychotherapist. We must hope that such first-aid as I can apply would help him to keep the symptoms within reasonable bounds.

I give two other examples of the sort of thing that takes place in these interviews because, although in practice they take up very little time and may seem of little importance, they do appear to have a valuable influence.

The first concerns Frankie Fox, of whom mention has already been made. Frankie (aged 13) was a boy of normal intelligence who had little interest in academic studies, but was an exceptionally keen nature student. He had an extraordinary " way " with animals and nature lore was a never-failing source of interest to him. He was a most pronounced individualist, finding difficulty in mixing

* Over 70 and nearly blind, my mother still retains her sense of fun and scorn of false dignity. She will not mind my broadcasting this silly incident.

happily with the rest of the community, but beyond that had given hitherto relatively little trouble. It seemed likely that he would grow up an oddity—a " character," but would find some sort of not too unsatisfactory adjustment. Unfortunately his younger brother Alec was highly intelligent and a good scholar. He passed the secondary school entrance examination and won a bursary. It was about this time that Frankie became really difficult. He became anti-social instead of merely a-social, and began to do a good deal of stealing. I made an opportunity to talk to him about the way our educational system tends to " glorify " the academic type of mind because the people who run it tend to have that type of mind themselves, and explained to him that there are other equally valuable types of mind which, while they may not be appreciated or exploited by our educational system, do often find appreciation in the world at large. I spoke of artists, administrators, leaders, and of various other kinds of specially gifted people who might be quite devoid of the capacity to pass examinations, yet able to do things which the most brilliant scholar may not be able to do if he lived to be a thousand. And I made it quite clear that he was in some such category. I wondered whether it was all so much waste of breath, but one day a visitor twitted him gently about still being at the primary school when his young brother was at the secondary. He replied, to the astonishment and amusement of the visitor, " I haven't got the academic type of mind. I've got another kind. Mr. Wills says there are other kinds of minds just as good as academic minds." I am not going to say that from that moment Frankie's troubles were over. But there was considerable improvement, and Frankie became a positive asset to the place before he left at fourteen to take a job at a zoo. Unfortunately, he was still too much of an individualist to keep this eminently suitable job, but it seems likely that he will find his level before long.

My other illustration also concerns two brothers. Cecil Bryant was nine when he came to Barns. He had been a persistent truant, had done some stealing, and was subject to temper tantrums. After about a year at Barns all seemed to be going well. There was much less stealing and fewer tantrums. Then came the news that his young brother was to come to Barns. He seemed worried about this, wrote to his mother warning her against it, said he was going to do his best to stop wee Harry coming to " this dump." When asked why he didn't want Harry to enjoy the amenities from which he had derived such great benefit and happiness (or words to that effect), he would break out into a tirade against " this dump," saying he wouldn't like his wee brother to go through all that he had had to go through, and so forth. However, Harry came in due course and Cecil immediately constituted himself his brother's protector. To the uninformed and superficial observer it was very charming to see Cecil " doing the big brother." But as Harry was quite capable of taking care of himself and, in any case, being very popular, needed no taking care of, it was to say the least, rather odd. Cecil would imagine assaults and insult of which Harry was quite unaware, and at the same time his own conduct deteriorated. He began to steal more than he had ever stolen, and his tantrums returned. It was clear that Cecil was consumed with jealousy of Harry, but was trying to compensate for these unacceptable feelings by his attitude of protection—just as Jacob Everson had to run away home to see if his mother was all right. His stealing was rather pathetic—he really seemed to take the most elaborate pains to try and get found out, presumably (though this is guesswork) in the hope of being punished and thus assuaging the guilt he felt for his wicked feelings about his brother. I let it all run on until Cecil himself seemed to realise that things were not going with him as well as they had, and then I suggested that he came and had a chat with me once a week. Weekly talks, which are exceptional, last for twenty minutes instead of ten. We make a regular appointment for, it might be, Wednesdays at 7.30. At 7.30 I am in my room ready. If the boy comes, well and good. If not, I do not send for him because normally I do not want to create the feeling that he *must* come. But afterwards I make a point of saying, " you didn't turn up at 7.30," so as to register the fact that I wanted him, and missed him. As long as the boy needs the talks and is getting anything from them he will not forget. When he starts forgetting they are usually discontinued.

Cecil and I then, talked inconsequentially for a week or two of this and that and then—apparently equally inconsequentially—I started telling stories about various people I had known. In due time I came round to someone in a similar position to Cecil (without of course drawing the comparison)—someone who was jealous of his younger brother. Then I told how this feeling can come about, how it can lead to difficulties if one tries to pretend it isn't there, how once one recognises its presence and realises it is a natural feeling one can cope with it. I deliberately made this a " serial story," knowing that if a bell were rung (so to speak) Cecil would want more next week, but that if he didn't want more next week, there would be no point in going on with it. But a bell was rung all right. When I enquired casually next time what we had been talking about last week Cecil had it all in detail and was anxious for more. So eventually I did apply it to his own case.

This, it seems to me, is the furthest the layman ought to go in the interpretation of symptoms. It was abundantly obvious that Cecil *was* jealous of his little brother, and it is only when a thing is obvious beyond any shadow of doubt that I venture as a rule to act on it. It is my fixed rule not to take positive action on a theory that is no more than a theory, unless we are absolutely stumped for something to do, and something urgently needs to be done. In that case the action based on theory must be of a kind which, if the theory is wrong, cannot possibly have any harmful effects. This condition, too, was fulfilled in the case of the Bryants, because if Cecil had not been jealous of his little brother it is highly improbable that the story would have made any impression on him ; and if it had made no impression it would not have been continued. I may add that the talks had an extraordinarily good effect on Cecil. The improvement in his general demeanour was most marked, and the stealing and tantrums stopped straight away.

So we chat away—sometimes with a particular end in view, sometimes with only the general aim of providing the feeling of being cared for ; sometimes we merely have a quick game of chess. There is an important particular in which my practice differs from that of the psychotherapist—it is no part of my aim to maintain the attitude of friendly reserve which the psychotherapist finds essential. In very many cases the children I am talking to have been denied affection and I, therefore, do not hesitate to shew it ; as often as not the interview takes place with the boy sitting on my knee. However much a boy may be embarrassed by that sort of thing in public (and that is all a matter of upbringing) the position is quite different when there is no one else about. The casual visitor to Barns may think us rather a sloppy lot with our kissing and cuddling and terms of endearment. There is much more of that sort of thing at Barns than you will find in any modern edition of Dotheboys Hall, but no more than you will find in any decent family—and we are taking the place, in many cases, of the family.

When the boy leaves my room I listen for his footsteps up the three wooden stairs outside and they are generally the light, hurried steps of someone who is excitedly pleased with himself. Though to be sure they might equally well be the light, hurried footsteps of someone who is jolly glad to have escaped at last !

The five minutes' gap between visits serves two purposes. It more or less eliminates the embarrassment of the second boy arriving before the first has gone, and it gives me time to make a few notes of what has transpired on a special sheet in the boy's dossier. The dossier contains two such sheets of " serial " notes, of which these are seen by no one but me, while the others are notes made at staff meetings.

Staff meetings take place once a week after supper, and all the staff attend. By all the staff I mean everybody—not merely, as some institutions would mean by that phrase, the teaching and administrative staff. Our staff meeting is for all the adults, though I have to admit that there might be difficulties about this if our domestic staff were not such exceptional people. But exceptional people or not, they have the same opportunities as anyone else of observing the boys, and they see very often a side that is hidden from the rest of us. So they all come, and we discuss half-a-dozen boys each week (in alphabetical order) so that each boy comes up for discussion every six weeks or so—making allowance for occasional times when Staff meetings cannot be held. Discussion begins by my reading over such social history as we may have, and the boys' personal particulars (age, I.Q. etc.), and then the Staff meeting notes from the time of his arrival—unless by mutual consent we feel it to be unnecessary in any given case. Then we just chat, and I make notes. Occasionally—though not very often—we have nothing to record but S.F., which means Steadily Forward. But it is only very rarely that there is nothing to record—of his attitude to so and so, an office he holds or has just resigned, his progress or lack of it in school, an interesting remark, a change in symptoms or progress of symptom for better or for worse. Sometimes we merely record such things as these, though sometimes there are also recommendations as to something that might be done or said by somebody or specific treatment to be tried, even if it is only a worm powder. He is to get some " extra attention " from so and so ; he is to be encouraged to resign a job that might prove too much for him, before he becomes too discouraged ; a new method of curing enuresis is to be tried ; the I.Q. is questioned and he is to be given another test. (We once found that the I.Q. of a boy which was said by the referring authority to be 92, was, in fact, only 77 !) and so on. Often there are conflicting views expressed (and recorded) and the meeting rarely finishes before midnight.

I give a specimen sheet of staff notes, which is necessarily rather a colourless one in order that the boy may not be recognised. He is the " President " of Chapter One.

Richard Smith. Date of Birth—1929. I.Q. 96. Admitted to Barns 12.12.194-.

12.12.4-. Sturdy little tough, looks as if he might have been a nuisance by reason of high spirits—sense of fun might have got him into trouble. Likes school (he says !) (W.D.W.).

30.12.4–. Full of beans and mischief, but apart from reluctance to wash, no outstanding symptom.

16.1.4–. Only one of his batch who did not bunk. Tore up some of his clothes, saying, " Why shouldn't I . . . they're my own ! "

6.2.4–. Diction and vocabulary very bad, always sounds truculent. R.W. (see below for meanings of abbreviations and initials) thinks he always looks worried. Frankly says he doesn't want to go home—would much rather be here. Always damaging boots, maliciously. His father is a bootmaker. An aggressive manner, J.P. says he was always very offensive and aggressive with her, kicking and spitting at her. Now much changed, becoming affectionate, takes her hand, fetches her a chair, etc. Arithmetic good enough for him to be in charge of " dippy " section, but English extremely backward (T.). Not aggressive with other boys—never appears at Committee. Quite keen on school (T.).

13.3.4–. A very happy boy now. Still looks worried (R.W.)—due to lack of vocabulary and faulty diction ? No reluctance to wash now.

24.4.4–. A very happy, attractive, cheerful little boy, though very upset by unkindness, real or imagined. Speaks a good deal at House-meetings. Singing lessons might help his diction (J.W.). A great storer of junk beneath the mattress. Some wet nightshirts lately. Says he did once wet the bed.

12.6.4–. A cherub (K.R.). Nothing to add to above except to note his refusal to accept bullying from Alf. Blake. Very backward in school, but very happy.

23.7.4–. During last two weeks has seemed unstable, less happy. Badly needs object of affection (A.H.). At present seems to need to hate everyone except love object of moment (W.D.W.). Says he dislikes R.W., but doesn't know why. This all seems to date from time of J.P. going on holiday and K.R. leaving.

6.11.4–. Relapsed considerably during A.H.'s stay here—perhaps associated with K.R.'s departure ? Very thick with and loyal to A. Blake, to whom, however, he is a rival for Janet's affections. Always wants to do things his own way—" I'll only do *this* much " (B.S.). Wants May to stay at 25 till he's 25 so he can marry her. Definitely seems unstable now, and face in repose is worried again.

8.1.4–. Very much under A. Blake's influence. Perhaps a little progress since last note, but still tends to bluster, etc. Went home at Xmas to stay with Granny, which he looked forward to and appreciated very much. Went to see his father while at home, but declined an invitation to stay there.

13.2.4–. Seems somewhat more stable. A keen and loyal member of C.A. A good committee man, with flashes of intelligence. Suggested that Jack McKay, who was rebelling against C.A., should be invited to meetings to see that their work was in his own interest. Quietly happy instead of boisterous (R.W.). Purposeful (J.W.).

19.3.4–. Treasurer of C.A. Now very friendly with Wally Straight, even to the extent of sulking when W.S. sulks, but in general happy and purposeful. Rather a pest at table, but only high spirits. Still very reluctant to say " please."

22.4.4–. Was Chairman of C.A. for a week, and then resigned following a row with Wills. Now Treasurer again. Father said to have " joined up or something," but has a nice lady looking after the house who says Dick can come home whenever he likes. Rather odd that he cannot read in view of relatively high I.Q. Wills to talk to him about this and suggest extra tuition with B.S.

27.5.4.–. Extra tuition suggestion rejected. Self-righteous wee laddie. Loves to be made a fuss of. Now much as he was last spring, happy, &c., but more mature with it. Went home to see his mother at Easter. She has " taken him up " and gets upset if he doesn't write, though she never wrote him once until a month or two ago. (Parents are separated)

1.7.4–. Mrs. Smith came on visiting Sunday with a man whom he called Uncle, but told other boys he was his father. K.R. (on visit) sees more decided change in him than in any other boy. Still his ebullient ·cheerfulness, but with more stable foundation. . An Elder.

19.8.4–. After being involved in trouble with J. Everson, W. Straight and Ted Bounce (while Wills away) asked for suspension from C.A., for a month and a " keeper." Was suspended for a fortnight and given K.R. as keeper. Above due only to high spirits—desire for a keeper really desire for a rest from responsibility (K.R.). Misses father-figure (W.D.W.).

28.10.4–. Now in Ben's class. Perhaps overcoming his reluctance to read. Still a trifle bumptious, but very little. Gang-leader of Torbank. Conscientious and keen. Happy and purposeful. Extraordinarily good at looking after Jack McKay.

2.12.4 . S.F. Very kind and helpful (M.F.). A very conscientious gang-leader and officer-on-duty. Vice-Chairman. Reads very badly, and takes the line that he won't rather than he can't.

28.1.4–. Reading difficulty now largely overcome. No longer refuses to believe he can read, and is making great progress. Was elected Chairman under new regime, but resigned following criticism from Wills and is now very happily Minister of Money. Dr. might be spoken to about adenoids.

3.3.4–. Rapid improvement in reading. No trouble. A happy purposeful child. Growing confidence in self, but will not attend Wyn's reading class if good readers are there. Very good at dealing in a sensible and friendly way with difficult boys. Still happily Minister of Money.

27.4.4–. Dr. says adenoid condition O.K. When Frankie Fox (Prime Minister) left, was elected P.M., and is doing very well. Extraordinary power of heart intelligence (J.W.). Returned from Easter holidays very friendly with everyone and pleased with himself.

17.6.4–. Now Minister of Work, but so conscientious that he has made himself very unpopular with other boys. . Was later sacked and generally " framed " by Paul Johnson (P.M.). P.J. admits having framed him. Wills wrote him a letter while away, and has had a talk with P.J. who admits his spiteful feelings towards D.S. Somewhat happier since getting Wills' letter, and is reinstated as Minister of Work.

18.8.4–. S.F. Inclined to bully a little. Much more confidence in himself. Wants to go on a farm, which is a good thing as it would not be good for him to go home.

20.10.4–. Due to leave at end of term. Great deal of malicious bullying in Wills' absence. Wills to see him to-morrow. He wants to go on same farm as A Blake.

17.11.4–. Now President, and a very good one. Very thick now with P. Johnson. We can see much improvement in this boy. His outstanding feature is his strong capacity for sympathy which, howeve rarely goes so far as to get him involved in serious misdemeanours with others, however much he may feel with them.   Is at present either displacing•some resentment against parents on staff, or is doing so in sympathy with P. Johnson.   There is every reason to hope he may do well, as he is fundamentally " good," though rather dependent at present on father-figure—a situation which would be met in a suitable farm job where he would live in.

    8.1.4–.   Went to a farm job, 2.1.4–.

In making these notes we sometimes record the initials of the persons making a particular comment, and these initials are given in brackets.   There is no need to give them in full, but I should perhaps explain that C.A. means Citizens' Association, and is not the initials of a person !   T. is Ben's predecessor, " Keepers" and " Elders " are roughly what their names imply. Torbank is the name of a dormitory.   The five dormitories are named after local hills—Meldon, Cademuir, Glenrath, Torbank and Whitelaw. S.F. means " Steadily forward "—a little domestic joke.

So much for the Staff Meetings.   But there exists another means by which a boy's progress is watched over, though it has existed, alas, more in theory than in practice up to now.   I refer to the Advisory Committee on Treatment.

It is my firm conviction that no such institution as Barns should presume to carry on its work without psychological supervision, though war circumstances have compelled us very largely to do so. Our Advisory Committee, of which we once had great hopes, consists of a Medical Psychologist, an Educational Psychologist, the Physician who normally attends the boys, the Social Worker, the Head-teacher and myself.   It began to meet once every six weeks or so, going through a few cases each time in much the same way as the Staff Meeting.   After two or three meetings, alas, it seems to have succumbed to the difficulties of war-time travel, and increased demands nearer home, though we still hope it is not dead, but sleepeth.   I find the lack of such psychological supervision a very grave handicap, and would not in normal circumstances tolerate it.

CHAPTER EIGHT

RELIGION

"I saluted the brave Scotch merchant . . . . and taking him by the hand I said to him : ' Blessed be God, we are once again among Christians.' He smiled, and answered : ' Do not rejoice too soon.' "

DANIEL DEFOE—" Robinson Crusoe."

I AM a Quaker, and what I have tried to do at Barns has been done in that particular way because I am a Quaker.

In saying this I do not commit my fellow members of the Society of Friends to agreement with this method or with my views, because Quakerism is not a set of dogma or a creed, and my Quakerism may differ from another person's. Many Friends find that Quakerism leadss them to pacifism ; some feel it their duty to serve in the armed force . I mention this only to illustrate how widely different interpretations of Quakerism may diverge, so that the reader may not assume that what follows is necessarily typical of the Society of Friends.

Although Friends have no creed or dogma, there are certain beliefs which have a very wide currency among them. One of these, perhaps one of the most important and widely held, is the belief in " That of God in every man." This is something more than mere conscience. It is, if you will, the breath that God breathed into Adam ; it is Browning's " spark " that " disturbs our clod " ; it is Whitman's " seed perfection " which nestles within us. This of God within us—to adopt another metaphor—is like water in that it perpetually seeks its own level, in which we may either help or hinder it. If we " give it its head," as George Fox and John Woolman, and many others have done, it may lead us into many strange courses, but our lives will be rich and purposeful, because they are guided by Him who guides the stars in their courses and whom we believe to have a purpose in the universe, though we have only the most fitful glimpses of what that purpose is. But while now we see through a glass darkly, we believe that when all men walk by the light that is within them, then indeed we shall see light.

It is this belief that has maintained an essential unity in our Society in spite of its lack of creed and dogma—that has, indeed, made them unnecessary; it is this belief, falteringly practised as it is here haltingly expressed, which has been the mainspring of our work at Barns.

If another man's actions seem to me to be evil, it must be for one of two reasons—either *he* is not following the promptings of the Holy Spirit—or *I* am not. If he claims that what he does is due to the guidance of that of God within him, then I must examine my own position with great care, and I must be most considerate in my dealings with him. Hence the sympathy of the Quaker for those who resist the demands of the State for conscience's sake. This is not due, as many may think, to the fact that so many Friends in time of war feel it right to resist the State's demands ; indeed Friends' expressions of sympathy with such persons would be stronger if fewer of their own people were involved. It is simply that they cannot feel it right to resist the promptings of God in another man, little as they may be able to understand those promptings. In such a case obviously—for the Quaker—any kind of harshness or coercion is out of the question. But what of the man whose ways seem evil, and who makes no such claim, who may indeed scoff at any such idea ? What should be our attitude to him ?

We cannot fail, it seems to me, to condemn what we know to be wrong, but it is not for us to condemn the wrong-doer. What we must do is to appeal to " that of God " that is in him, and try to get him to look inward to the springs of his conduct in the hope that he may find a worthier motive than those that have hitherto led him. I claim no novelty for this attitude. It is one with which many people, both now and in the past, would agree. The question is, how is this particular approach to be put into actual practice ?

The founders of what has come to be known as " the Pennsylvania System " had much the same approach, and it led them to a method which some of the least humanitarian among us to-day would condemn. They put all their criminals in separate cells in a specially constructed building, with absolutely no communion with each other and the minimum of contact with anyone else. The theory was that the compulsory meditation and self-communion thus imposed would cause the prisoner in time to see the wickedness of his way—even perhaps to find his way to the Light Within—and lead him in time to the stool of repentance. In fact, as we now know, it made him bitter and resentful, and he spent his time cogitating on the wrongs that had been done to him, instead of those he had done to others—unless indeed he became quite insane.

Here, however, I must insert a parenthetical explanation. There may be those who are by now accusing me of confusing those two entirely different concepts, " crime," and " sin," which, they will say, are by no means the same thing ; while it may be our duty to be tender-hearted and forgiving to those who sin against God and us (and who may or may not have broken a law) we are not necessarily committed to such an attitude in the case of those who have broken a law—and who may or may not have sinned. I confess that this always seems to me sheer casuistry. Truly, the terms sinner and criminal are not synonymous ; but they are in a large degrèe co-extensive. There are at the one end those who have " sinned " by, *e.g.*, committing adultery, or by robbing the poor and fatherless by methods technically legal, and who are not criminals ; at the other end are those who commit " crimes " by failing to fill in a form required of them by the State, or by refusing Military Service, but who cannot on that account be called " sinners." But between these two extremes is the common run of burglars, cut-throats, brigands, bandits, and what you will, whose offences are both criminal and sinful. Am I to have two attitudes to such persons —one as an individual and another as a citizen ? I find that very difficult—especially as this is supposed to be a Christian State—and it seems to me that our attitude, whether as citizens or as individuals, should be based on the teachings of Him whom we claim to follow.

If then (to revert) we want people to see that of God in themselves, the best and most obvious way to help them, it seems to me, is to let them see God made manifest in other people. As Christians we believe that God is love, and I have failed badly in what I have written up to now if I have not made it clear that it is just love that has been lacking in the lives of so many of the people who start life like the boys of whom I am writing here, and who grow up to be called criminals.

It seems presumptuous and very far from humble in us to claim that what we are trying to do is to shew forth God not only with our lips but in our lives ; and He knows how miserably we fail. But that *is* what we have got to try to do, just because it has so rarely been done in the case of the children in our care. We must so conduct ourselves that they will come to see in us something they have hitherto not known, and which it is no sin to covet for themselves. They must be loved in order that they may learn to love. That is not only Christian teaching ; it is sound modern psychology.

How then in particular is this love to be expressed ? It is difficult (though not so difficult as those might think who have never tried it !) to " turn on " love at will to all and sundry ; but at least we can try to cultivate a loving attitude. We have explicit instructions about this—" Do good to them that despitefully use you " ; " Love your enemies " ; " Be not overcome of evil, but overcome evil with good." I cannot feel that I am overcoming evil with good if I coerce a boy by means of corporal punishment—or any other kind of punishment—however successful it may at the moment appear. This is the " other reason " referred to in Chapter Two for the non-use of punishment at Barns. If punishment overcomes evil at all (which I do not for one moment believe) it has overcome it with evil, as I cannot believe that the deliberate infliction of pain for the sake of inflicting pain (and not incidentally and unwillingly, as in the case of, *e.g.*, pulling out a tooth) is anything but evil.

It is true that there must be order, there must be some measure of discipline, there must be a respected authority even in a small community of forty persons. That I do not attempt to deny. But in order that there may be the minimum of misunderstanding and resentment, let us, so far as possible, make such rules as may be necessary *between us*, so that the need for and the occasion of them may be seen by everybody ; and if breaches of these rules should, occur, let us also deal with those *between us*, for the same reason. It may be found necessary for the common good—or even for the good of the individuals concerned, to prevent worse befalling them —to restrict the liberty of some, which may seem very much like punishing them. But if the decision is arrived at as the result of a discussion among his peers, he may at least understand the reason for it. It may even be that the community—consisting as it does very largely of persons holding beliefs other than those of which I have been speaking—may come to inflict some mild penalties, as indeed they have at Barns. But at any rate that helps them to learn how futile (if they do not know already !) and unfriendly punishment is. I have known boys restrict the liberty of their own friends, for his own good or for the good of all. They are very much more reluctant to inflict upon a personal friend a penalty that is purely punitive. The orthodox may say that this indicates a very poor sense of duty. To me it indicates that to the uncomplicated and severely logical mind of the child, punishment is incompatible with love.

Men are not necessarily aware of the Inner Light which burns within them, and it is obvious that we who believe in its presence in all men must be extremely careful in our dealings with others lest we make it more difficult for them to discover it ; lest we do anything to hinder its growth or make it difficult for men to follow its promptings. This is one reason why we are so extremely reluctant to do violence, physical or intellectual, to another's person. This is what leads us to be tolerant of many things which we should perhaps consider wrong for ourselves, and obviously it involves a passionate belief in freedom, for it is only in freedom that there can be real growth. I have given already several reasons why we at Barns believe in the maximum amount of freedom for the boys in our care. They were for the most part reasons based on a rational judgment of what was most likely to be helpful in contributing to " the therapy of the dis-social," but the underlying and fundamental reason—for me—is, as with the non-use of punishment, a religious one. I believe this was true of Homer Lane in his work at the Little Commonwealth, and frankly I very much doubt whether it is possible to carry on such a regime unless one's methods have a spiritual origin. I know that there are many " progressive " schools, run by professed rationalists, in which there is as much freedom and as little punishment as at Barns, and there is even one well-known school, the head of which is not ashamed to use the word love. But these are Boarding Schools where the children live only for part of the year, the rest being spent in the respectable middle-class homes from which the children came, and in which—however difficult and neurotic the children may be—there is some kind of home background, and at least some training in the social graces. With us it is different. The children are with us practically all the time, and the training they had before they came to us is, one is sometimes tempted to think, worse than none at all. There are times when we seem to be doing no useful work at all, when a boy upon whom we have set the highest hopes will do something that seems to suggest we have never touched him, times when the whole business seems so discouraging as to be hardly worth-while ; times even when we feel that we should like to scream. If, at those times, our work was based *only* on rational grounds, we should begin to doubt its value, and I very much doubt whether I could keep on with it. But because we are able to say with T. S. Eliot (however unscientifically !) " Take no thought of the harvest, but only of proper sowing "*, I am able to carry on.

This is one reason why I find it very difficult to argue with the orthodox. The orthodox will assess results, and if these do not seem good will say : " There's something wrong with your methods." When I assess results (so far as they can be assessed) and find them doubtful, I say, "we have not applied the method properly," for we base our methods upon "what we have received" and not upon what the results seem to be. This is highly unscientific and improper; but it is, I venture to think, with all humility, the kind of obstinacy that has made for much progress, in many fields, in the past.

So much, then (and perhaps too much) for my own religious attitude and the religion underlying our work. But what of religious teaching ?

When I, as a conscientious objector, appeared before a Tribunal, I was asked whether I taught pacifism to the boys at Barns. My reply was that I hoped so, and as I watched the several eyebrows

* In " The Rock."

of the Tribunal rising in unison, I explained that as my whole work and my attitude to the boys were based on the religious beliefs from which my pacifism springs, I hoped the boys would in time tend towards that religion as a result of having seen it in action but that the deliberate inculcation of pacifist doctrine would be; contrary to what I conceived to be sound educational principles.

If ever there was a pious hope (in any sense of the phrase you like !) that seems to have been one, because I see very little sign of any Barns boy inclining towards my particular brand of religion. But that again is due to my faulty exposition of it, and I must try to do better. Not that I really look for immediate results ; our boys are already abnormal enough without adding the abnormality (as it would be, in a boy of 12) of piety ! But I do devoutly hope that in later years some at least of our boys, when they reach the age at which people begin to think about religion, may say to themselves, " Those people at Barns had something—I must try to find out what it was."

That, then, as I have implied earlier, we are presumptuous enough to regard as our main religious teaching, and there are many people who might think there should be no more than that. But in fact we do indulge in some religious teaching by word of mouth also, and it seems to me that there are excellent reasons for this, even on purely " rational " grounds.

I had the great good fortune to be the son of pious parents. One of my earliest memories is of a highly illuminated text which hung on one of the walls of our home—" As for me and my house, we will serve the Lord." Even before I had learnt the story of the redoubtable old warrior and his errant and vacillating compatriots, I was impressed by the challenging and unequivocal ring of that statement. One felt that the next words ought to be " a.nd be damned to the lot o' ye " ; which indeed they were, in effect

If Joshua had belonged to a certain modern school of thought, he would never have delivered that magnificent harangue about God's mercies and the iniquities of " your fathers which were the other side of the flood," nor its grand climax—" Choose ye, therefore, whom ye will serve." He would have said something to this effect :—
" I have formed certain conclusions concerning the nature of the transcendental, which I propose to keep to myself. As for my house and all the rest of you—you can form your own conclusions too, but without the benefit of my experience and my opinions on the subject." In other words—" No, we don't tell them about God ; we want them to decide for themselves when they grow up."

How on earth—or in Heaven—can they " decide for themselves," if they never hear anything but the case for the opposition, which is all that they are likely to hear if the parents do nothing about it ?

I consider it of the utmost importance for their sense of security, that children should know exactly where their parents or parent-substitutes stand—though there should be no pressure on the children to take the same stand—and, therefore, in order to make it clear that we attach some importance to religious observances, my wife and I have carried over into the family life of Barns our private family practice of devotional readings in the morning and evening. I need hardly say that attendance is entirely voluntary ; it is not the Victorian kind of family prayers where everyone is compulsorily assembled, the servants standing in serried ranks, each according to his station. About half the boys attend, though the numbers vary a good deal. The evening reading was quite early on replaced by the singing of a hymn.

But this in itself creates further difficulties. It stamps me definitely as belonging to the vague general class of those who " believe in God " without saying very much about the God in question, and leaving the boys to assume that my God is the very unpleasant and vindictive tribal deity about whom they have heard from other sources. For I find that so far as our boys have any ideas about God at all, they are of the most primitive nature. They are not only crudely anthropomorphic, which is understandable in children, but God is conceived of, in the main, as an omnipresent, all-seeing monitor, who is setting down all their misdeeds against the day of reckoning. That beautiful image which Jesus used—" Our Father, which art in Heaven "—does not mean to them what it meant to Jesus. Very often it means—such is the nature of some fathers—something so very different that I have had to avoid its use. I often hear boys announcing, with great belligerency, " I dinna believe in God," or " God's all a lot of boloney." It was not the taking of His name in vain that worried me, and I should have been quite happy about it if I had been able to take it at its face value. But it could not be taken at its face value. I knew enough about those boys to realise that it did not mean " I have thought the matter over (or ' I have been convinced by my father's teachings on the subject ') and I have arrived at the conclusion that God is a myth." What it meant was that they were terribly frightened of this heathen God they had been brought up to believe in ; frightened not only of him, but of pretty well everything else, and in trying to prove to themselves and to others that they were really bold fellows, they said in effect, " *I'm* not frightened—not even of God ! " Some of my rationalist friends say that this is a good reason for

" cutting out " religion altogether in such a place as Barns.* It is associated in the boys' minds with fear, which we are trying to exorcise, and if you want to do away with the fear, you'd better kill the bogy-man.   But that is just what you cannot do.   I do not mean that you cannot kill the bogy-man because you cannot kill God.   That is not the point, because this bogy-man which they think of as God is not my God at all, and frankly you can do what you like with Him for all I care.   But the point is that the idea of the existence of this bogy-man, God, was implanted in their minds at such an early age (often by no other means than blasphemous references to His name) that it cannot be removed as easily as all that.   Far better, and easier—even on strictly rational grounds—admit his existence and say—" but He isn't like *that*— He is love, and all that that implies.   It is because of this God that we insist on you having ' your freedom,' and refuse to beat you or knock you about ; so He can't be so bad after all "—and perhaps after a while they'll stop being frightened of Him.

So it was necessary to find some means of dissociating myself from the false gods " which were the other side of the flood," and to take the fear out of the primitive theology held by the boys.   To do this I started a Sunday morning service, and here I must confess to having made a very serious mistake.   A mistake, not in the holding of the service, but in the measures taken concerning attendance. I said it was to be entirely voluntary—and then I did my best to get everyone to attend.   It is true that if a boy steadfastly refused to yield to my " moral persuasion " and was prepared to be unpleasant rather than attend—he usually stayed away.   But sometimes there *was* unpleasantness, and I have known occasions when I was in such an unchristian state of mind by the time the service was due to start that I have had to say so and dismiss the meeting.   So— although that sort of thing was very rare—it was an unhealthy sort of business, rather like the sort of thing one hears spoken of (falsely for all I know) in the Army—" A and B companies will parade at 6.30 sharp for a voluntary lecture."   But we had some lively discussions for all that, and sometimes the service was as hectic as the House-meeting.   I raised no objection ; indeed I welcomed criticism, and sometimes there was plenty of it, though I only remember one occasion when things became so completely disorderly that I had to ring down the curtain before we had reached the end.   That, then, was our Sunday service until the Citizens'

* Samuel Butler says in his " Notebooks "—" Theist and Atheist ; The fight between them has been whether God shall be called God, or whether he shall have some other name."   And, he might have added, between the various kinds of Theists, too !

Association started. Then—as the Citizens' Association was going to be responsible for all activities outside school—I asked them if they were making any arrangements for a Sunday service. They said " No," and made it quite clear that this was not merely due to an oversight. I asked if I might attend a meeting of the Association to give my views on the subject. They said I might, and when I went they listened very politely to all I had to say. Then they went to the length of voting again on a question which had already been decided, with the result that my eloquence was shown to have been useless. There was to be no Sunday service for the Citizens. Of course, there was nothing to prevent my starting a private show of my own for " as many as will," but I thought that would hardly be playing the game. So, having shot my bolt, I just waited to see would would happen next. I did not refer again to Sunday services, either publicly or privately, until three weeks later, and then the subject was not broached by me. The Chairman of the Citizens' Association came to me just as we were finishing breakfast on Sunday morning, and said : " If we have a service, will you take it ? " I grumbled about the short notice, but said I would. I was warned that it would be absolutely voluntary, but most of the boys turned up. I " took " this service, but suggested that in future they should give the speaker a little more notice. In future, however, the service was not " taken " by an adult. A Committee was appointed each week, which chose hymns and readings (with or without adult assistance), appointed readers and a chairman, and invited someone to speak. Usually it was an adult that told the " story," but quite often a boy would do it. And so the service continued until I was instrumental in killing it—or at any rate, until I caused it to lie down after it was dead. Some two years or so after the events I have just described, interest waned. Committee members, appointed to run the service, " forgot " to make the arrangements, or to turn up at the service, so things became very flat indeed. Then some difficulty was experienced in finding boys willing to serve on the Committee, so I suggested one week that as most people didn't seem to want to have a service, it was stupid to insist on trying to appoint a service committee each week, and those who wanted a service should be left to make their own arrangements. That was several weeks ago, and there hasn't been a service since then. But one of these days someone will say, " Why do we no' have a sairvice ? " and it will start up again.

CHAPTER NINE

EDUCATION

"We can polish him up by and by; and as for learning, he will pick that up as pigeons do peas. So don't hurry him."
LOUISA M. ALCOTT—" Little Men."

VERY little that the boys do at Barns may not be called education. When they are " playing about " in the river they are learning to swim ; when they are climbing trees, they are developing physical agility and several other qualities besides. I find it almost shocking that this altogether admirable and natural exercise is a *crime* to the city dweller. One boy who was taken from Barns against our advice was returned in a fortnight because—among other things— he had been brought home by an angry park-keeper who had found him climbing trees. What a remarkable civilisation it is in which a boy may not climb a tree !

The educative value of shared responsibility is obvious ; but that I have already dealt with. Restricting slightly the use of the word, I propose to devote three chapters to education. In the first I propose to speak of spare time activities, which I think of as the truest education, and one of the most important aspects of our work. In the second I hope to refer to ordinary schooling, and in the third, under the heading of re-education, I shall say something of the educational therapy carried on in the school.

Apart from pure pastimes like " hide and go seek " (as it is quaintly called in Scotland) and those dreadful spontaneous games which seem to consist largely of charging boisterously through the house, yelling wildly, and slamming all the doors as you go, our first spare-time activity—which has continued to be one of the most popular—was woodwork. A small room was furnished with a couple of old benches and some tools, and the boys were invited to use it on certain occasions when I could be present. It has never been thought of as a " class." I am only there to see that chisels are not used as screw-drivers or missiles, and that planes are not used to shave off the heads of nails. I may also—so far as I am able— give a little advice when asked.

I went to woodwork myself as a Council School boy. For years I had looked forward to the time when, proudly wearing my woodwork apron, I should be old enough to go to " manual," and at the age of eleven or so I started. I went once or twice a week for about eighteen months, and learnt only one thing—that I was

88

" no good at it "—which was false. I was told to plane a piece of wood until it was " square," and it was explained to me that as long as a crack of light could be seen between the try-square and the wood, it would not do. I took the instructor at his word, and I do not remember that I ever did anything else but try to remove this crack of light from successive pieces of wood. Twenty years later I started again with " Bunny " Barron, at Hawkspur Camp, where I learned that to get a piece of wood absolutely square as I had struggled to do at school, requires the skill that comes from years of practice and (equally astonishing !) that the correct way to hold a tool was the way that comes most naturally to you—provided it is a way unlikely to damage you, the tool, or your neighbours. Under Bunny's tuition I made great progress because in the usual sense of the word it was not tuition at all. One got on with the job, and if one got into difficulties Bunny was there to help one out. In eighteen days I acquired more skill and confidence in the use of tools than I acquired in eighteen months as a boy under tuition.

So that is the method we use at Barns. We are not out to make carpenters ; we are only out to make self-confident and self-reliant men. Most of the boys who come to Barns have, to a greater or lesser degree, a sense of inadequacy and failure. One of our most important jobs is to replace that feeling with one of achievement and self-confidence. A boy who can handle a joiner's tools with familiarity and ease is on the way to developing such a sense—and he may even become " pretty good at it " in the process. So if you go to woodwork at Barns you make what you like, any way you like, and if you like you can ask Wills for advice.

Most boys begin by making a sword. It is easy to make and useful to play with. (The horror of those woodwork classes where only " useful " things like egg-stands and pipe-racks are made ! To a child only those things are useful (broadly speaking) that can be *used* in play.) You just get a short bit of wood and nail it across a longer bit. The only snag is that if you ask Wills to lend you his knife to sharpen the end the old so-and-so will say, in his grumpy way, " Why borrow my knife when there's a row of perfectly good chisels in front of you ? " In due course (sometimes I warn them of this, sometimes I don't bother) the cross piece will come off, and that is the time to say, " It will stay on better if you joint it. But if you want to be chump enough to waste another nail on it you can "—then one can show how the halved joint is made. There are several books knocking around in the woodwork shop with ideas for making things—toy engines and motors (we made a fleet of them and, at the suggestion of one of the boys sent them down to the evacuated nursery school) dolls' cots, and so forth. In December woodwork will be full of boys, making Christmas presents for their brothers and sisters, often starting on them much too late to have any hope of finishing them in time. But if they are done in time, I can imagine them almost bursting with pride as they hand them over—" I made it masel'." There could be no better medicine for a boy who feels that his life, up to now, has been a bit of a flop. I shall shew in chapter eleven how woodwork kept Sammy Johnson from utter frustration until Ben could give him a sense of achievement in other spheres.

Generally speaking, if a job is done well enough for the boy, it is good enough for me, but I do sometimes encourage a boy who can do good work to acquire a sense of craftsmanship, and might even in such a case forbid him to take it from the shop until it was done in a way that we both recognise as " properly." But those occasions are rare.

That is not the whole of woodwork, however. There are the jobs that we do between us, for common use. In 1940–41 was first created that Barns Institution, " The Barry "—what Scouts would call a trek cart. We worked on it throughout the winter, and Ernest Ludlam got us some old motor-bike wheels, had them fixed on an iron frame, and the " barry " was done. Each successive winter or spring we took it to pieces and re-built it, usually because it had broken, owing to some defect in the structure—and there were often running repairs at camp, too—until by 1944 we had a really substantial article which, although rather heavy, did at least carry our goods to camp without giving way under the strain. The parallel bars, the various diving boards and rafts, have all been communal efforts, and as much satisfaction has been found in their making as in their use. Then there are jobs about the house. For many jobs of course we have to call in professional help, but many others are done by myself or one of my colleagues, assisted by a small gang of boys—broken tables, beds and chairs, door knobs, electric light switches, and so on, without number, have been mended in this way. There are very few boys who are not in a position to say, after a year or so, " *I* helped Willsy to mend that "—or, with even greater pride—" *I* mended that." I enjoy " fiddling about " with tools, but I should no more think of doing a small repair job by myself than Ben would think of teaching an empty class-room. I should feel that I was wasting my time.

The value of keeping a free-and-easy, spontaneous atmosphere in all spare-time activities was never more clearly shown than in our experience with gardening. Gardening started quite spontaneously, and at first was not even encouraged, because we were making plans for getting a piece of land ploughed up for this purpose later on. But the boys started digging up tiny little bits of the playing field, in the most disorderly and untidy way, and calling them gardens. As the playing field was quite useless, anyway, as a playing field, we said nothing about this, and as there was no damping the boys' enthusiasm we helped them, after a time, with seeds and advice when they asked for it. There were some twenty or so of these plots—some of them not more than a yard and a half square—but the enthusiasm was terrific, and was sustained from the spring well on into the winter. The following spring we tried to encourage those who wanted to do gardening to have their plots on the piece of land we had set aside for that purpose which—with a very bad grace—they did. But gardens were still scattered about without any kind of order or design, and the place was very untidy, though enthusiasm was still fairly high. The next spring I anticipated them by marking out with great care, several rows of neat square plots, and said, " anyone who wants a garden can have one of these." It practically killed all interest in gardening, and we have had to revert to the old untidiness, but we have never managed to recapture that first fine careless rapture.

There is one activity, however, in which interest never wanes and which is of tremendous value as an outlet for the emotions, as an expression of the fantasy-life and as an opportunity to do something creative. Here again—as with woodwork—the value is in the *doing* and not in the thing done. At painting we are not trying to make artists—but happy children, and thus satisfactory adults.

There are three kinds of painting activity, The first is imaginative painting in watercolours. Pots of brightly-coloured paint are placed down the middle of the tables, and those who want to paint (generally more than can be provided for) are given paper and brush and told to go ahead.* The enthusiasm and energy that go into this sedentary occupation are really astonishing.

A large number of the painters—whether consciously or not I am never sure—carry on a running commentary on their work all the time they are at it. " This is a giant and he's got a big stick in his hand. It's not a stick really it's a tree that he's pulled up " (on go the boughs and roots). " Here comes another giant, and this giant biffs him on the head with his stick—BONK " . . . Half-

* I find that this is much the same as the method used by Mrs. Marie Paneth at her "Branch Street " club. " Branch Street " is a most fascinating book (George Allen & Unwin Ltd.) the more so to me as it describes exactly the type of child that comes to Barns—though Mrs. Paneth's children were Londoners.

a-dozen boys might be chattering away like this, quite oblivious to everything and everyone except the world they are creating. It is fascinating to watch the imagination growing ; or to be more accurate, to watch the boys overcome their fear of giving it free expression. When Harry Bryant started, he would paint nothing but a witch's house, sometimes with and sometimes without, the witch flying over it on her broomstick. This went on for some weeks, until he had, so to speak, completely painted the old witch out of his system. He had been a frightened, furtive, vicious-tempered little boy, but now he began to learn how to smile. He started on a richly varied series of paintings of many kinds of subject—fairy stories, imaginary landscapes, historical scenes, stories that he " made up," houses, palaces, gardens, Barns episodes —and all with a vigour and clarity of line that was most effective. Presently—that is after a year or so—we found him drawing with a brush rather than painting, a series of types of person, each with appropriate headgear and background—a cowboy, a gangster, a Trojan, a Norman, a King, a beggar, and so on. There was one to which he gave no name, but which we have decided must be intended to represent a decadent of the nineties ! He also did a portrait sketch of me which, though far from flattering as a likeness, has much to recommend it as a picture. My background consists of a row of bookshelves on one side carrying a vase he remembers having seen in my sitting room ; and on the other a picture which he also remembers having seen there. He was not more than ten at this time.

This kind of painting is an interesting measure, too, of the degree to which an emotional conflict is getting straightened out, as well as having itself a useful cathartic value. Ginger Bright, who had been brought up by his Grannie, had an intense and openly expressed hatred of his mother. He had remarkable fantasies about killing her and these were mixed up in an extra-ordinary way with fantasies about Jesus on the Cross. His early paintings beggar description, both as to design and as to colour. They are an indescribable jumble of crosses, knives, daggers explosions, bombs, aeroplanes, all in the most lurid or the most sickly of colours. Week after week these dreadful monstrosities were produced but very slowly, as Ginger began to get rid of some of his resentment—in paint and in the many other ways provided at Barns—his paintings gradually began to be slightly more coherent in design and less horrific in content. Gordon Steel was a boy who had been separated from his parents at a very early age, and little was known about them except that they were highly undesirable. Gordon himself was very backward intellectually (I.Q. 73) and seemed at times almost unteachable. But he had a rich and vivid imagination, and a sure hand with the paint-brush. Some of his queens and princes and fairy kings (very popular subjects with these deprived children) were a delight to the eye. He never referred to his mother, but used to invent wonderful tales about his father, sometimes saying that he was dead and describing the heroic manner of his demise ; sometimes explaining that he was abroad, and telling wonderful tales of his exploits there. He had a strong sense of deprivation over this matter of having no parents to write to or to be visited by—but rarely mentioned his mother. One day he painted a large and horrible-looking face with tears streaming down it. He explained that it was a boy crying, because he had seen his mother !

In all this the rôle of the adult (usually my wife) is similar to mine at woodwork—to discourage the application of paint to other surfaces than that of the paper, and occasionally to give advice if asked. But less advice is given here than at woodwork. Ruth will never give in to a request to " tell us what to paint," and only in very exceptional circumstances will she give technical advice. To give advice is to imply that a child might be right who, from fear or from ignorance, says " I can't paint," and of course, such a child never is right. Any young child, unless discouraged by stupid adult teaching, can express himself in paint. But it must be borne in mind that young children's paintings are entirely different from those of older children or of adults, and are to be judged by entirely different standards. A child will be perfectly satisfied with something which may look to you and me like nothing on earth, and I presume this to be, because the child does not yet very clearly distinguish between what he has put on the paper and what he sees in his mind's eye. When he looks at the paper he is also looking at the mental picture he had formed and I expect that, taken together, they make a very satisfying sight. This does not prevent some young children from displaying a very good sense of design, of rhythm and of form, if only they are not interfered with by fussy adults trying to " teach " them.

But there does come a time when they need to be taught. The sort of paintings I have been speaking of are done in the main by the younger boys. As they get older they begin to separate the image from the picture ; they begin to criticise their work ; they want to know about perspective and other technical things—they want to paint a picture and not merely to express a fantasy. The age at which this stage is reached varies enormously in different children, but one of the most unfailing signs of its approach is when the child begins to join land and sky in an horizon. The young child (very logically, as it seems to me) bounds his picture not only round the sides, but at the back also. His painting does not go as far back as the horizon, so there is a gap of white paper between earth and sky. One day (and Ruth always feels it to be rather a sad day) he will produce a picture where the muddy brown of the earth meets the rich blue of the sky across the middle of the background—and you know he is beginning to grow up.

Then Ruth starts him on oils, and here we have to acknowledge our great indebtedness to our own teacher. Arthur Segal died only this year, and though, happily, his work is being carried on by his daughter, his death was felt as a very real loss to all who had worked with him. Here again, with Arthur Segal, I learned as a man what they had failed to teach me at school—that it is possible even for me to paint ! " Everyone," said Segal " can learn to paint," and if you looked incredulous (as I did) he would add in his somewhat explosive English (for he was a Roumanian and never became a fluent English speaker) " I zhall zhow you." Ruth and I took him at his word when he said that, and when war circumstances brought us to within twenty miles of his studio we took to spending our weekly day off there. We had considered ourselves—as so many do—congenitally incapable of painting a picture, and our going to Segal was rather in the nature of a challenge. We had seen him do remarkable things with other people, but had always said—as perhaps some of my readers may now be saying, " But *he* couldn't have been as bad as *us*." We were simply astonished and I, at least, was filled for a time with a wild enthusiasm at what we found ourselves able to do after half-a-dozen lessons. Unfortunately (from that point of view), we moved North after a couple of months, so tuition stopped. Unless one is Winston Churchill, one cannot do everything so, Segal's point having been demonstrated, I let painting drop, but Ruth kept it up so far as her busy life has allowed. I cannot describe nor expound Segal's method—a description of a method is bound to be more or less a comparison with other methods, and I know no other method. I cannot say how I started learning to paint any more than I could say how I started learning to talk, and I don't think Ruth can either—except that the method is based on the fundamental assumption that of course, everyone can learn to paint.* And it is obvious that, consciously or not, when Ruth

* See also the quite independent, but really astonishing work done among epileptic children by my friend, Charles Handley Read, and described by him in " The Studio," March, 1944.

starts teaching she will reproduce the methods that were used so successfully on her. Not with the same skill, nor the same background of knowledge, nor with the same consciousness of direction ; but the general approach will be the Segal approach.

Here there is one extremely important point to be noted. You do not need to be a brilliant artist yourself in order to get other people—children at any rate—to paint. The principal qualifications are enthusiasm and a conviction that there is no-one who cannot learn. I am glad to have had this view confirmed by someone who knows much more about it than I can ever hope to know. Since I started writing this book, Mr. Herbert Read has published his " Education through Art," which no-one should miss who is interested in education or in art. I did not find it an easy book to read, and it is not cheap, but I am glad to have spared both the effort and the money ! In preparing this book, Mr. Read apparently visited a large number of schools and one of the things that impressed him (p. 288) is that the best work does not necessarily come from the schools that are best equipped with materials or with technical qualifications. The best work is the result of a relationship between teacher and pupil that is quite independent of these things.

So oil painting (" taken " by Ruth) has been the second form of painting, with very interesting and encouraging results. The boys are very keen to do portraits, so Ruth puts them on what is probably the most difficult, but certainly the most interesting form of portraiture—they paint themselves. To this they bring great enthusiasm, industry and concentration, and there is one very important and interesting thing I have noticed about the results, namely, that however bad a likeness a boy may paint, he always manages somehow to reproduce—sometimes in a most striking way—a face that displays some of the salient features of his character, or of his mood at the time. So marked has this been that I have thought it worth while to reproduce some of these paintings to help the reader to form an impression of the sort of person about whom I am writing. Although they are excellent character studies they are very poor likenesses, and cannot be recognised by friends and relations !

Not that oil painting consists, by any means, merely of self-portraits. There is the usual range of subjects, some indoor and some outdoor ; usually chosen by Ruth, but sometimes chosen by the boy himself. Sometimes a boy who was not very successful in watercolours will do well in oils, because oil-painting is much more disciplined than the other kind, and he may feel the need of discipline ; and of course, conversely. Though there are some happy people who are naturally deft, and these will shine in either form. Some of these clever people I find extremely irritating. Ian Burns was such a one. His I.Q. was 77, but he was singularly clever with his hands. He could come to woodwork and handle all the tools as if he had had years of experience. The first time he came to oil-painting he painted as if he had been at it for years. His products at hand-work and clay modelling are superior to most people's. And does all this mean anything to Ian? Not a bit. One might have been forgiven for hoping that this was one of those cases (by no means as frequent as is often supposed) where intellectual inadequacy is compensated by manual dexterity, but it is not. The lack of intelligence is there, the skilful fingers are there; but the one by no means compensates the other, because he seems quite unaware that his work is good. Indeed he does not often take part in any of these activities except by persuasion— they just mean nothing to him at all, and what the answer to that is, I have not yet discovered.

As a half-way house between the two forms of painting I have referred to we have experimented a little with the method of Cizek which is described in Viola's book, " Child Art." The children are told a story and are then asked to paint it. I have not yet found this to have valuable results, but it is only in its early days as I write.

It is impossible of course, to deal with all the various occupations that go on at Barns at the same length as I have dealt with those to which I have already referred. Nor is it necessary to do so, for the general atmosphere that I have tried to describe is the same whatever is being done, the general method does not vary greatly according to the subject. The first essential is the spirit of freedom about it all—you can please yourself whether you go or not, and when you get there you can please yourself within certain limits what you do. Then there is the sense of achievement, which in some cases needs no encouragement, but which in others needs to be induced by means of praise. I have heard people whose attitude is much the same as my own say that they never give anything *but* praise. I think that is going rather far, but it is essential that nearly every-thing should be praised for something or other. A child who already has a tendency to feel inferior will easily convince himself that his work is poor, but will greedily lap up praise (though sometimes seeming to spurn it) and by it be encouraged to do something else and earn more praise—all the time adding to his skill and confidence and lessening his sense of inferiority. Praise is essential, and so is enthusiasm in the teacher. An ounce of enthusiasm is worth a ton of technical knowledge, and that is not hyperbole; it is not even

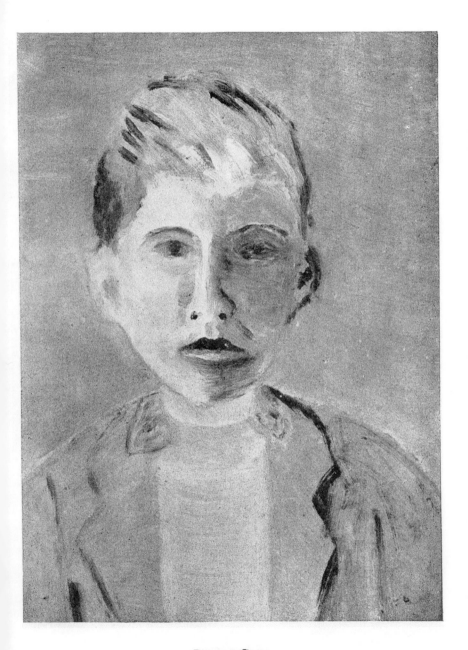

DANIEL GOFF
Self portrait

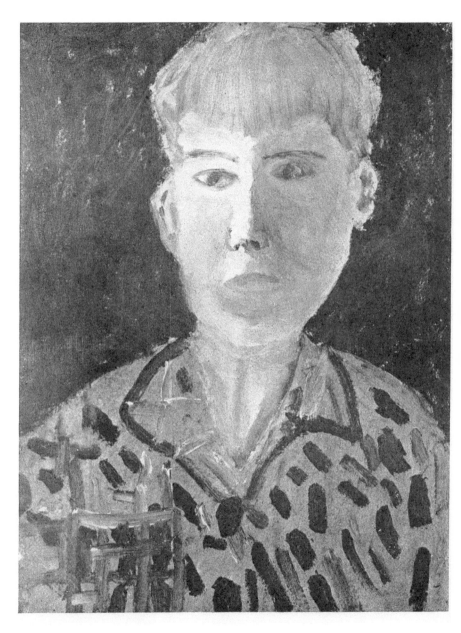

ARTHUR COLLINS
Self portrait

exaggeration. Where there is enthusiasm and ignorance, teacher and boys can learn together. Where the teacher has knowledge but no enthusiasm little that is worth learning will be taught. Indeed if it were possible, which, of course it is not, I think it would be an excellent thing if the teacher could start each term as ignorant or almost as ignorant as his pupils, in the subject he is to teach. The first winter he was at Barns, Ben had most of the staff playing recorders, and the boys were encouraged to make bamboo pipes, which they then painted and learned to play. Squeaking and whistling were to be heard in all parts of the house at all times of the day and night, and it was difficult to judge whether the boys or adults were the more excited about it all. Some of the boys even saved up their coppers and bought themselves recorders. The staff practised assiduously every night after supper, some items for the Christmas concert, but when we solemnly took our places on the stage and raised our flutes to our lips, the audience thought it excruciatingly funny. We had barely finished the first of our pieces when Bobby Dodd cried out, " You lot get down now, and let us have a go " !

The percussion band, too, was very popular, though I found that this was a case where the teacher really does need to know more than the pupils. I discovered that when I tried to " take " percussion !

Clay modelling, too, has been a very useful activity, having much the same value as painting, and into which a tremendous amount of energy goes. Then we have done weaving, soft-toy making, making chess-men out of old cotton reels, lino-cutting and printing—and so on and so on and so on.

These are all activities in which the children *do* something, and it is very desirable that most of a child's programme, should involve him in some form of activity. But many of them have passive corollaries. The keen painters may sometimes be found in my sitting-room looking—under Ruth's guidance—through our books of reproductions of paintings. Sometimes there are gramophone recitals, and it is sheer nonsense to say that children do not like good music. Much depends upon how it is presented to them. Most of our gramophone recitals take place when the boys are in bed, during that useful period between going to bed and going to sleep. Sometimes a story will be told or read, sometimes there is some poetry, sometimes there is nothing, and sometimes there is wireless or a gramophone recital. It is well known that children tend to be rather conservative, and those who have never heard anything but dance music prefer to stick to what they know. The answer to that is to get them to know something else, and the chances are that they will like that as well. So I get them into bed (or the Officer on Duty gets them into bed, to be precise) and with a great show of enthusiasm promise them a great treat—the Concerto Grosso of Handel, or a Beethoven Quartet. The boys with no experience of this kind of music will emit mock groans, but others will be quite glad to lie in bed and listen. I might say a few words about the music or about the composer while I am winding up. the gramophone. Bach's large family is a never failing source of interest. For one reason or another we have not been doing so much of that lately (at least I haven't—though they may have been getting it from someone else) but when I was doing more of it we reached a stage where pieces would be asked for by name. The third Brandenburg was a very popular choice, and they loved to wind up with a two piano version of " Sheep may safely graze." There is much excitement when, as sometimes happens, " our " music is heard on the wireless.*

And much the same applies to poetry—there is no need to dwell on it—if it is presented by someone who is enthusiastic about it he will communicate his enthusiasm. If it is presented by a stale teacher who regards it as just another subject, no good will be done to anyone.

All this sort of thing (and there is much more of it than I have mentioned ; I have not referred to play-acting, to camping, to nature-lore, to mention three important things) is the real education, and that is why I have called the next chapter " Schooling." The acquisition of and drilling in mere technical skill—in reading and writing and counting, are of course, essential preliminaries ; but they are not education.

---

* Not that we deprive them of their " swing " music ; God forbid. It has its place, but is not allowed to exceed that place.

CHAPTER TEN

SCHOOLING

" Meditating on the Situation of Schools in our Provinces, my Mind hath, a times, been affected with Sorrow."

JOHN WOOLMAN—Writings.

ONE Thursday in November, 1942, there was great excitement at Barns. A few weeks previously I had asked His Majesty's Inspector of Schools to pay us a visit as he had not been since, two years before, he had told me that we were a case for " the larger charity " ; and here he was.

It was Ben's day off, which meant that his group—the older boys—were working in their room entirely unattended, though it is true that the Head and *his* group were next door. I had a talk with the H.M.I. (wondering furiously what was going on in Ben's room !) and then directed him to the school hut. Then I returned to my own room to await his return. He was away for well over an hour, and when he came back he told me something of what had happened. They were (I was relieved and perhaps a little surprised to hear) all working away industriously, and he gathered them round the fire for a chat. He asked them what sort of things they did, looked at their books, and then talked to them about themselves (" I am sorry not to have seen Mr. Stoddard, but it was obvious to me that some very good work was being done there"). To Frankie Fox he said, " I remember you from the last time I came. You and some more boys were in a room with Mr. Wills writing a letter to your mothers about your having run away a few days previously. Do you ever run away now ? " " Oh, no ! " said Frankie promptly, " we always ask Mr. Wills if we want to go home now." This was a lie, because Frankie was still apt to take French leave occasionally, and I told the H.M.I. so. I did this, not so much because I did not want the inspector to be deceived, as because I thought Frankie's loyalty was a more useful argument in our favour than Frankie's apparent probity. He wouldn't, two years earlier, have told a lie just in order to give an inspector a good impression of Barns School. And thereby hangs a long and, I hope, an interesting tale. The change in Frankie's attitude to school—and of all the other boys, for that matter—was almost entirely the work of Ben, than whom no man ever had a more

loyal, a more enthusiastic, or a more tireless colleague. He wrote
a good deal of what follows, and where quotation marks are used
with no explanation, I am quoting from a long paper he wrote
at my request.

Before proceeding with the story, however, I must make one thing
clear. If I had my way, attendance at classes in such a place as
Barns would, I think, be voluntary. As I do not have my way there
is no need to dwell at length on that—I merely mention it to explain
what might seem an inconsistency. Barns is an Evacuation Hostel,
and its inmates live there by reason of their being pupils at an L.E.A.
school. Voluntary classes would mean a large number of noughts
in the register during the early days of a boy's school career, and it
is very doubtful whether the authority would be satisfied with the
explanation that lessons are voluntary. Indeed, in so far as I am
in loco parentis and " my " children are pupils at an L.E.A. school,
I have (apparently) a statutory obligation to see that they attend.
We have never attempted to escape this obligation in its entirety,
because we were already asking the authorities to stomach rather a
good deal, and we did not want to seem too impossibly cranky.
So we have just said to the boys that whether we or they like it or not,
the law compels them to go to school.

Having made that point clear, we may proceed to a little history.
When Barns started we had one teacher, appointed by the
Edinburgh Education Authority. We have called him Teacher,
or the Head teacher, because we cannot tell the tale without
bringing him in, and we cannot bring him in without causing
the sympathetic reader (if there be one) to regard him somewhat
unfavourably. This is not because he is an incompetent or an
unsuccessful teacher ; he is neither of those. His only failing
would by many be considered a virtue—he did not wholly share
our point of view. And as I am necessarily writing from our point
of view . . . but I will stress this no further. As soon as I heard
that he had been appointed I wrote to the L.E.A. and told them
that in spite of his obvious good qualities I feared he would in time
find the atmosphere here unhelpful, and would complain that the
methods adopted by the rest of us made the maintenance of
discipline in school difficult or impossible. Which, in fact, he did
at the end of the first term.

I have already told how his visit to the Education Office brought
us a visit of a sub-committee of the Education Authority ; but it
brought us other things as well. It brought us the strap—the belt,
as they call it in Scotland. The teacher had, hitherto, tried to avoid
the use of corporal punishment in school, but after his visit to the

Education Office he gave up the attempt. I did not, and do not, feel that I could blame him. He had thirty unruly boys to teach, whose mental ages ranged from about six to about 14, whose unruliness was undoubtedly, during that trying first term, exacerbated by the way we treated them out of school hours. And the very fact that our outlook was different, made it difficult for the rest of us in our limited free time—to lend him a hand, quite apart from the fact that he did not feel easy about making use of unqualified assistants in work which was primarily his responsibility.

However, the time came when we were able to provide him with more material help than an odd hour or two, now and then. In the summer of 1941 Kenneth Roberton, our first sub-warden, left us to take a joint appointment with his wife. Kenneth was a great loss to us, and his outlook was so similar to my own that his presence in the first few difficult months immensely lightened my own load. But by the time he left, things had become much less difficult, and we, therefore, decided that his successor should be a qualified teacher, devoting half his time to teaching, and the other half to helping in the supervision of the boys out of school hours. The L.E.A. agreed to this appointment of a half-time teacher, and in October, 1941, with their approval, we appointed Mr. Benjamin Stoddard, B.A., a young man who had been dismissed from his first teaching post because he was a conscientious objector. Ben, like myself, is an integral pacifist. That is to say, his pacifism is not merely a reluctance to be a soldier, but is an attitude to life. He had been given unconditional exemption from military service under the first conscription act, before the war started. He therefore, had no difficulty in adapting himself to the Barns way of doing things, but the fact that he was serving two masters—Teacher and me— did not make things any easier for him. He was given a group of the younger boys to teach in the mornings, and from the first tried to avoid the use of an authoritarian attitude—with difficulties that can easily be imagined. But the birth of the Citizens' Association early in 1942 changed all that.

I have told of the birth of the Citizens' Association in Chapter Five, and on page 54 I referred (in a letter to our Chairman) to " an interesting bit of backwash " in the school. In short, a little rebellion took place. It started with truanting, and the ringleaders seemed to be the very boys who had been largely responsible for the formation of the Citizens' Association. I was at first—until I grasped its import—perturbed by this, and at dinner-time one day began to harangue them. They said they were having a rebellion. " Are you rebelling against me ? " I asked. No, they were not. " Against the adults generally then ? " No, not against them. They were rebelling against the Teacher. " But my dear fools," I said (or words to that effect) " In the eyes of the law I am the person responsible for seeing that you go to school, so you are rebelling against me. In so far as I have shared that responsibility with the Citizens' Association, you're rebelling against yourselves as well. If the Teacher wanted to be unpleasant he could go to the authorities and say, ' Things have come to such a pretty pass at Barns now that they can't even get the boys to school,' and I don't see what good that would do anyone—though I do not for one moment imagine that he *would* be so unpleasant." But whatever the Teacher's attitude might be, the fact remained that in the eyes of the law I, and I alone, was responsible for getting them to school, and rebellion that took the form of truanting was therefore a rebellion against me. There was silence for a moment or two while this fact sunk in, then Frankie Fox enquired, with a wicked little twinkle, " Is it anything to do with you what happens when we get to school ? " I said that I was naturally interested in their schooling, but technically it was outside my province. After that they went to school, and though some of them may have absented themselves after having once got there, others remained in school to make themselves as unpleasant as they could to the Teacher.

I need hardly say that in this they received no encouragement o any kind from me or any of my colleagues, but I should be worse than a hypocrite if I pretended that the boys did not realise that we sympathised with their end, whatever we may have thought about their means. Teacher did not hesitate to use his strap, but he quickly realised that this was something more than passing insubordination, and that it would take a good deal of strapping to quell it. I am sure he could have quelled it if he had laid on often enough and heavily enough, but it is to his credit that he saw the futility of that, and came for a talk with me about it. I told him quite frankly that I thought the new regime in the house was largely responsible for the trouble he was having in school, and Ben and he and I, and Mrs. Smith who happened to be visiting, had a discussion about the whole thing. The upshot of it was that the older boys—about ten of them—were handed entirely over to Ben. Officially, Ben was only a teacher in the mornings, took his free time in the afternoons, and returned to duty in the evenings. This meant that the rest of us had to teach his class for the short afternoon session. We gave them woodwork, poetry, painting, handwork and what-not—in short we undertook to keep them constructively occupied. The idea was that this group should be entirely shut off from the rest, and should be brought within the ambit of Shared Responsibility. The position would be, in effect, that the Citizens' Association would run its own little school, with Ben and the rest of us as teachers.

Thus it came about that on Monday, 16th February, 1942, we began—after eighteen months—to bring the school into line with the house. It was an exciting time, but we were not by any means jubilant. Ben says " Of the ·first morning's school I remember chiefly a sense of dismal failure and an almost overwhelming feeling that circumstances were going to be too much for us." " The Citizens made themselves responsible for discipline in the school as they had in the house, but not at first with the same success. An Officer on Duty was elected by the Citizens (changing daily) to maintain order in the group. If necessary he was to bring charges for disorder or non-completion of work, before the Committee which met daily." It didn't seem very successful at first. They were all generally retarded educationally, most of them with specific backwardness in one or more of the basic subjects. They must all have spent several years at school frustrated, neglected, always at the tail end, attempting work which was too difficult and in which they could take no interest. Small wonder that they seized their first opportunity to work off some of their resentment against the institution associated with their unhappy experiences.

" In the absence of imposed discipline therefore, they assumed that they were free to do as little as they liked, and were unwilling to organise themselves or discipline those who came in late or refused to do their work. The crux of the matter was that these boys were not convinced when we said ' Your group is not like ordinary school. If you do your work, it will not be because you are bullied into it, but because you are interested in it and want to get on.' " For, of course, they were *not* interested, and they soon made that plain. But Ben had the answer, as will be seen. " I believe that in those early days our sincerity and conviction were on trial. Situations arose every day which put to the test our decision to refrain from all coercive discipline. The boys were trying to find out just how far they could go ; they were seeking to prove whether we meant what we said or not." They had proved that we meant it in the House, but that was a different matter. Living in an Institution was a new thing to most of them, so they were prepared to find new ways. But School they knew all about. School is a place, as they knew from experience, where you do as you're told, do it smartly, and no back answers. School is a place where a man (or woman) armed with a strap compels you to do meaningless things for no apparent reason.   This thing here is called school, so it must really be the same as all the others.   " From daily refusals to do work, daily complaints that they were bored, daily requests for something more interesting and of more use when they left school, it was clear to me that both curriculum and teaching methods would have to be adapted to the new situation.   Fortunately, the practical activities provided by the rest of the staff in the afternoons were greatly appreciated by the boys and kept the scheme going for the first few days.   After a time I was able to give the schoolwork a more practical bias, insisting continually on the everyday usefulness of the things we learned.   We counted money, did shopping sums, calculated wages ; we measured tables, windows, rooms and made plans to scale of all kinds of familiar objects.   We wrote letters, read exciting stories, acted plays, talked about things we had done or hoped to do.   A good deal of field work in nature study was done," much of the instruction being given by Frankie Fox, who knew more about birds and beasts and their habits than the rest of Barns put together, men, women and children, " and we discovered a wealth of wild flowers and river and wood life.   The Committee of Management arranged excursions to historic Edinburgh and these did much to associate the new schooling with happy and interesting life as distinct from the unrelated perplexities which had hitherto aroused so much antagonism.

"One or two of the older boys began to ask me for individual work in their weak subjects, so that when they left school they would at least be able to meet ordinary situations.   I, therefore, gave them assignments in those subjects, at which they could work, not only in the official school hours but at other times as well. Out of this arose a modified form of the sub-Dalton Plan, by which there were weekly assignments in each subject, and freedom to arrange work according to individual needs.   A balanced minimum of work was required and a weekly meeting of the group was held —sometimes attended by David Wills—at which each week's work was considered.   A report of this meeting was presented to the Citizens' Association and any necessary action was decided on then. If, for example, a boy still had work to finish, this was discussed at the class meeting, and reported to the Association," which may or may not instruct him to finish it over the week-end.   Usually they were told to finish it, and usually they did.

Ben had his day off on Thursdays, and on those days I used to attend school to answer questions and advise or help as necessary. I was not there as teacher, much less as disciplinarian.   Even so, they resented my presence after a time, and had me removed. This simple thing made a big difference—they were really convinced that we were in earnest, a better spirit prevailed, and Thursday mornings passed—very often—industriously and quietly. It was to this group, on such a Thursday, that the Inspector came, as recounted at the beginning of this chapter.

The Citizens' Association never managed this group as well as it did the rest of the house, partly because it was just a group, with the contradiction of the rest of the school still there, but outside its jurisdiction. Not every boy appreciated freedom from repressive discipline, for there is quite a good deal of superficial security to be found in it, and some boys are quite at a loss when it is removed. But it is probably true to say that whatever serenity and purposefulness was achieved was largely due to the new satisfaction the boys were finding in their work.

So school continued until the end of that year (1942) when the Head teacher left. At last the period of divided loyalties and conflicting methods was ended, and the change in the atmosphere —especially in school—was all that we had hoped.

But it was a tough time for Ben, because for the first five months he was single-handed in the school. He very wisely refused from the start to attempt to teach all the boys at once, and the L.E.A. sanctioned, as a temporary measure, the "half-time" school for which, in 1940, permission had been refused. To the teacher accustomed to teaching 30, 40 or even 50 children at once (if teaching be the right word for it), 30 may not seem an impossibly large number for a class. But the mental ages of our boys ranged now from 6 to 16, quite apart from the fact that they were at Barns because they were "difficult." Schoolwork was therefore, divided into two kinds—basic subjects and the rest. Ben looked after the basic subjects by taking the boys in two shifts of three hours each, morning and afternoon. This was all the official schooling there was, and nothing else was called "school" in talking to the boys. But we also provided a very wide range of "non basic" subjects at all hours of the day and evening, including week-ends, for any who were not in school. We all took a hand in this—cooks, cleaners, House-matron, as well as Ruth and I—even Ben found time to make a contribution to this side of the work, in addition to his six hours a day solid teaching. It meant that Ben and I had practically no "time off" (apart from our weekly day, which we never surrender) for nearly five months, but we both felt it to be well worth-while. The participation of the boys in this non-academic work was absolutely voluntary. There was no pressure to attend, but the classes were offered rather as a privilege than as a duty, and they were very well attended. We had the ambitious aim of having each boy attending classes voluntarily for ten hours in the week, thus making up the ten of which he was being deprived by " half-time school," but in this we were not quite successful. It would have been rather surprising if we had been, because we normally limited the classes to six boys, and all the classes had to be done in the free time of the adult in charge, or while he was doing something else. Nevertheless, several boys exceeded the ten hours we hoped for, and the average for the 30 boys was between 7 and 8 hours each week. Of course, education cannot be reckoned in hours, but we wanted to convince the official mind (if necessary) that very little was being lost as a result of " half-time school."

We had been prepared for another increment of disorder when the last shackles of imposed discipline were removed but, although some boys were unsettled and were manifestly pining for the heavy hand, Ben's unfailing patience and the influence of the steadier boys kept it within much smaller limits than we had been prepared for. There was a little truanting, some fooling in the class-room, and that sort of thing. But anything which interfered with the smooth working of the school was reported by the Officer on Duty to the Committee, and dealt with by the pressure of public opinion, which was definitely against disorder. They wanted to see " our school " succeeding. And in spite of many difficulties which even then had not been foreseen—succeed it did.

CHAPTER ELEVEN

RE-EDUCATION

"Suaviter in modo ; fortiter in re."
Quoted (too often) by LORD CHESTERFIELD to his long-suffering son.

GORDON STEEL was an enthusiastic painter. Every time there was painting, Gordon was there, and we often had difficulty in dragging him away from his paint-pots when it was bed-time. One day— for a reason I do not remember—Ruth took painting during school hours, instead of during the evening. "Is this school ? " asked Gordon. He was told that it was school. " Oh, well, I shall choose something easy to paint, so's I can get out early ! "

This beautifully illustrates the general attitude to school when Ben took it over, and which he set himself to reverse. First the reasons for it had to be found. One had already been found and dealt with—the system of repressive discipline under which most schools are run. If this is good for any boy—which I deny—it is certainly not good for Barns boys, so it was done away with and the School, as I have shewn, was brought within the range of Shared Responsibility.

This did not produce any magical change because the prejudice against school and the pre-conceived idea of a teacher as a man with a strap are so deeply embedded. If you watch any group of children playing at school, you will find that it consists very largely of the " teacher " administering corporal punishment to the children. What a tribute to the teaching profession !

But very gradually a change was brought about. A year after Ben took over he happened to refer to himself as the teacher, and received the retort from one of the smaller boys, " Garn—you're no' a teacher ; you're just a man " ! What a tribute to Ben ! The Teacher had come down off his pedestal and had become a human being.

I do not suggest that the abolition of repressive discipline will of itself do away with the antipathy to school, but it is a much more important thing than many people realise. It is difficult to learn anything from a person whom you dislike or of whom you are frightened ; learning from those we love is a pleasure. I know that your ordinary disciplinarian will say that his boys do not dislike him, and of course a boy has his degrees of likes and dislikes even among the disciplinarians of his environment. But in general it is the kind, affectionate teacher, rather than the stern and unbending disciplinarian who is liked by his pupils ; and it is *that* kind of teacher who, other things being equal, will get the most work out of his children. During my own short school career, I was top of each succeeding class until I entered the class of a teacher with a very bad reputation, of whom I was terrified, when I sank quickly down to the middle. Even though all children may not re-act as violently as I did, it is obvious that such a teacher is not getting the best out of his class—yet the fools think they are efficient because " you can hear a pin drop " in their class-rooms. This confusing of good discipline with good teaching has gone on too long, and it is surely time it was done away with. So great is the prejudice against a little noise in the class-room that even Ben has sometimes wondered whether our class-rooms were not too noisy for good work to be going on. When he had examined the statistical evidence of the first year's work he wondered no more. But I anticipate.

It is true of course that a boy—unless there is something wrong with him—admires virility, and that is often particularly true of the sort of boy who comes to Barns. The trouble is that most of them have been brought up to regard physical violence as the highest manifestation of this masculine quality, which sometimes causes them to *admire* even a man who knocks them about, and of course they will seek to emulate him. It is our job to provide them with a different standard.

They will hate school then because of the way it is conducted. A child is a bundle of energy, and his school work should involve him in as much activity as possible. Activity moreover, that is designed to give him a sense of achievement, to make him feel that he is *doing* something that means something. The dull daily round of mechanical processes stimulates no interest, gives no sense of achievement, and produces boredom and worse. Then they get behind with their work, much of what the teacher is saying becomes incomprehensible to them—and they just stop listening. They thus become quite lost, settle down at the bottom of the class, where they are bored, or lost in fantasy, or frustrated and angry, according to their temperament. This, of course, is one of the evils of big classes. The teacher must address himself to the mass, and the " special cases " simply have to be neglected.

Where backwardness is due to defective intelligence of course no really curative method is possible, but it is possible to arrange that the less intelligent are not taught at the same time and in the same way as the more intelligent, and that the two types are not brought into competition with one another. I believe that this problem is beginning to be tackled by most Education Authorities, by the use of " three stream " or other methods. Nevertheless, we do get at Barns a number of boys whose difficulties have been largely contributed to by this factor, and for them the only remedy is careful, painstaking and patient individual attention in which—and this is the vital point—their achievements are measured by comparison with their own previous standards, and not with the achievements of their more intelligent contemporaries. To say—or even to imply—" Johnny can multiply in £.s.d., but Tommy at the same age can't even do simple addition " is damning. But to say, " Well done, Tommy ! Last year you could only add two lots of figures and now you can add six "—that is the way to encourage progress. That is Ben's way. To allow them to come into competition with brighter boys is to create a feeling of inferiority which may cause great unhappiness, emotional problems and an inhibition of effort. Only yesterday Bobby Dodd, our very successful Chairman, refused to take an attainments test. He is a boy with a fine personality, a born leader, and popular with everyone. But his I.Q. is not very high, and in spite of our efforts to avoid a competitive spirit, he was afraid' that it might appear that he was not as " good " as some boys—though of course he did not give that as his reason.

Then there are the boys who have " got behind " by missing school. Sometimes this is unavoidable, as in the case of Sammy Johnson. But even so, the results in unhappiness and frustration leading to violent anti-social conduct outside school as well as in it may be serious.

Sammy arrived at Barns when he was not yet nine, and this is the first note we made about him :—

" Arrived a poor-looking, frail, downtrodden frightened thing, furtive and pathetic. But with, nevertheless, great capacity for mischief, ' devilment,' disobedience, mulishness, tantrums and every other kind of ' wickedness.' Language deplorable as to vocabulary, subject-matter and diction, which is very childish. Has a good working knowledge of the ' facts of life ' and gives expression to very adult sexual fantasies. Always joins any truanting party. A knife-thrower. A biter and scratcher. Very responsive to affection."

He had already been absent from school for half his school life as the result of accidents and illnesses. When he had been at Barns about three months he had another serious accident which resulted in his being in hospital, off and on, for another year. When Ben took over the school Sammy was 11 years old and practically illiterate. He shewed a very strong sense of inferiority, bursting into fits of passionate anger and tears whenever the question of his reading came up. He loathed books, and for a long time either refused to have anything to do with reading, or at best approached it with a studied indifference. When asked to do a piece of work his immediate cry would be " I'm not going to do it. You won't get me to do it. Nothing will make me do it." This obstinate refusal to do work was of course a cloak—for the benefit of the other boys—of his inability to do it, or his fear that he might not be able to do it. Much better distinguish oneself by making a scene, than make oneself look silly by being unable to read a simple thing that the smallest boy can read ! His fixed attitude to reading overflowed, unhappily not only to all English subjects, but to the rest of his school work. His attainments in arithmetic were nearly normal, but when faced with a new piece of work, even before attempting it, he would say, " I canna dae it ; it's too hard ! " This in a voice full of pent up emotion, fear, frustration, defeat. And then, unless one was prepared to devote the rest of the lesson to him, there were behaviour difficulties, inattention, fooling and bullying, ending in tears.

While Ben was making a frontal attack on this difficult position others of us were making an outflanking movement. We thought that if we could find some sphere of activity in which Sammy could distinguish himself, it might enhance his self-confidence, and make him less unwilling to admit deficiencies in another sphere. We therefore fostered his faint interest in woodwork until it became his principal occupation outside school hours, and one only had to mention woodwork to think of Sammy. He was now, I must say, very good at it ; but he very soon thought he was, and we put him " in charge " of the woodwork ,ope. He was also at this time, " Minister of Routine," and the refrained, so far as possible, from criticism of the not very sfficient way he carried out his duties, because they gave him a good deal of compensation.

Ben, once he had got things sorted out, started a special class in the afternoons for boys needing therapeutic work in the schoolroom, hoping that all those who needed to come would do so voluntarily. In the main, they did ; but not Sammy. He was encouraged, then persuaded, then urged, and perhaps in the end even nagged—for the problem was becoming urgent ; Barns boys leave school at 14 ! But Sammy was not going to take the step of openly

admitting that he needed " extra school." One day, during a rather
warm argument with Ben on this subject, he said " You canna make
me go to extra school." This was a very broad hint, and Ben took
it. It meant—undoubtedly—" I should like to enjoy the advantages
of extra school, but cannot do so without losing face—to go voluntarily is to admit that I'm not as good as I might be at school-
work. If, however, I were compelled to go, no such admission
and, therefore, no such loss of face would be involved." " Oh,
can't I ? " said Ben. " Well—from now on you go to extra school,
whether you like it or not." This was, strictly speaking, quite
unconstitutional, and if Sammy had liked to challenge him at
Committee there's no knowing what might have happened. The
very fact that he did not charge Ben for wrongfully compelling him
to go to extra school was a clear justification for Ben's action.
Sammy made a show of protesting, sometimes had to be hunted up
at extra school-time ; sometimes even had to be carried struggling
to school, but the struggles were not very thorough, being intended
purely for the benefit of the onlookers. After a few days Ben
abandoned the idea of having Sammy at ordinary extra school,
and had him, instead, in his own room (and his own time !)
but before six months had elapsed Sammy was asking to be
allowed to go to ordinary extra school. His self-confidence was
increased, he was calmer, had fewer " paddies," and gradually
began to lose his interest in woodwork—he no longer needed
it. Sammy is far from cured—but a very good start has been
made.

Sammy, it is true, is an exceptional case in that the absences
were involuntary. But it does show what can be the result of
" getting behind " in school.

Many others have been absent voluntarily—the truants. Most
Barns boys have truanted a good deal at one time or another ;
Harry Bryant, for example. He was nine when he came to us.
He was of normal intelligence, but had put in only one third of the
possible attendances during his first three years at school. His
reading was equivalent to that of a boy of 6, his spelling to that of
a boy of 5. His history is a picture of aggressiveness and destructive-
ness—" Will attack anyone and will return to the attack some
time after being dragged away "—" Had a phase in which he was
continually smashing things."—" Intense fantasy life—paints
furiously and gets very excited over it." His home circumstances
were such as I may not dwell on here ; sufficient may be gathered
from what I have to say in Chapter 13. A boy with this kind of
background and temperament stays away from school because he

doesn't like it—the regimentation and the unimaginativeness of routine school-work in a class of 40 or so is just intolerable to such a person. Then, of course, he gets behind in his work, which causes exasperation in him as well as in the teacher—and so on.

Much could be written about the reasons for truanting, but they all come into three main categories—those arising in the school, those in the boy himself, and those arising in the home. Of course, I speak now, not of the occasional truanting such as we all enjoyed from time to time, but of persistent truanting over a long period of time. And of course all my three groups of causes inter-act upon one another. School seems an unpleasant place— so one stays away. That seems to me a very natural thing to do, and the reasons it may seem unpleasant I have already given. Or one might stay away because one doesn't get there in time. It would be silly to tell the teacher that, but it is what happens in many cases, of which Ginger Bright is only one. His father is said to have died when he was a baby, and his Grannie brought him up while his mother went to work. He developed what seemed to be an intense hatred of his mother, and indulged in extraordinary fantasies in which he stabbed her or drowned her, and did away with her in all manner of unpleasant ways. Sometimes these day-dreams would make him so unhappy that he would escape into an entirely different kind, in which he was an explorer, or was living the natural life of the birds and beasts of the woods. His fantasy-life was so absorbing that he would become quite lost to the world, and would " wake-up " in the middle of the morning to the fact that he was still on his way to school. It is easy to see how he would become " backward " and a school-hater. This was the boy, who, when his mother re-married and took him home said : " I'll go home, but I won't go to school ; I'm coming back here to go to Benjie's school." And he did, too.

Then there is the group of reasons associated with the home— slovenliness, lack of order and method, lack of interest in the children—all of which militate against regular school attendance, besides creating emotional problems tending to inhibit interest in school-work, leading to backwardness, truanting, and ʳo round the vicious circle. An extract from the social worker's notes on Walter Scott will illustrate what I mean. " . . . family consists of father, mother, Walter aged 10½, and other children aged seven, six, and two . . . House consisting of two rooms, was in a dreadful condition of filth and untidiness . . . Girl of seven was pale and wan, and obviously not in good health. Headmaster of School says the

family is very bad—no discipline—father was lazy. Had been
told to take children to the clinic for scabies treatment, but had
refused to do so. Girl of seven had suffered so much with scabies
she hadn't been to school for six months . . . Attendance Officers
were never out of the house . . . father had been fined ten
shillings because of Walter's repeated absences, but it seemed to
have no effect on him . . . " I quote this not as the worst
example, but merely as the first that comes to mind, and it is
fairly typical of this type of family. No-one cares two hoots
whether you go to school, or what you do with your time. So
why bother?

So backwardness may be caused by the nature of the school
regime, by limited intelligence, by involuntary absences or by
truanting. But there are other causes. You might be a fairly
regular attender and still do badly if your emotional life is not
happily adjusted ; but as I have already amply illustrated that sort of
thing, I will say no more about it.

There remain the physical causes of backwardness. One
immediately thinks of bad sight of course, with its obvious remedy
of glasses. But mortality of glasses is so high among our boys that most
of them are without more often than they are with them. I was
thinking, however, rather of a more subtle kind of physical disability.
In fact, I am not sure that it is physical. Perhaps we should do well
to borrow that very useful phrase from McDougall's famous definition
of an instinct, and call it psycho-physical, thus offending no-one.
I refer to the phenomenon known as " Left Laterality." It means
that the person concerned is left-handed or left-eyed or both. This
may not seem a very dreadful thing, but it may seriously affect
learning capacity because the left-lateral person has a tendency to
move from right to left when you and I would move from left to right.
Such a person very easily gets into difficulties with his reading and
writing, and its repeatedly making apparently stupid mistakes
such as spelling words backwards, or reading them as if they had
been written backwards. And not only in English, for there are
many mechanical processes in arithmetic in which one may become
hopelessly muddled if one gets one's sense of direction mixed up.
We were, therefore, not surprised to discover (more precisely, to
have discovered for us*) that about two-thirds of the boys resident
at Barns had one or more of the symptoms of this characteristic,
and Ben had to set about finding the best way of coping with it,
for it requires very special teaching methods.

* By Dr. M. MacMeeken, M.A., B.Ed., Ph.D., who has done a great deal of
research in this field.

These, then, were the boys with whom Ben had to deal. School-haters who had never had any interest in their school-work, had never had any sense of achievement, who had experienced in their school lives nothing but exasperation, frustration and defeat. And who were therefore, nearly all backward.

He first set himself the task of discovering the *degree* of each boy's backwardness, which he did by means of attainments tests.* These test a child's attainments in much the same way as the intelligence tests discover his capacity. As intelligence tests give a " Mental Age " so attainments tests give an " age " for reading, spelling, or whatever the subject might be for which the test was applied. If, for example, a boy of ten can read only as well as a boy of eight might be expected to read, we say his reading age is eight ; and just as we can get an " Intelligence Quotient " by the formula

$$\frac{\text{Mental Age}}{\text{Chronological Age}} \times 100,$$ so we can get a " Quotient " for each

subject tested by the analogous formula

$$\frac{\text{Reading (or whatever it might be) Age}}{\text{Chronological Age}} \times 100.$$

The use of quotients is convenient because it removes the need to look up each boy's age every time one considers his attainments. The layman will probably think of them as percentages, and although this is heavily frowned on by the experts it does help the uninitiated to see what it is all about. The Attainment Quotient of a boy who is normal will be 100, if he is bright or dull it will be above or below 100 accordingly. Below, then, are the results of the Attainments Tests, which Ben applied in Reading, Spelling and Arithmetic, and I ask you not to follow my frequent practice of skipping the figures and going on with the text. Instead of giving names and ages I have given I.Q.'s, which enable you to see at a glance how retarded a boy is—one would expect his Attainments Quotient to be somewhere near his I.Q.

* The tests used were :—
> For Reading—Burt's Re-arranged Word Reading Test, published by The Scottish Council for Research in Education.
> For Spelling—Spelling Test, by the same Council.
> For Arithmetic—Burt's Tests in the four fundamental operations.

These tests are useful, not only in assessing attainments, but also in discovering special weaknesses and individual difficulties. Especially useful in this connection, too, were Prof. Schonell's carefully graded tests in Arithmetic.

Intelligence Quotient	Attainment Quotient in		
	Reading	Spelling	Arithmetic
71	62	61	45
72	78	65	90
75	79	70	73
77	64	59	61
78	56	58	58
78	111	102	90
78	70	66	74
85	81	80	88
85	55	50	74
86	60	60	Infant level
88	105	97	76
89	90	77	61
89	82	71	73
89	78	71	58
93	94	78	61
95	93	90	?
96	64	56	67
96	104	91	76
97	92	80	63
97	67	62	60
97	124	102	77
98	98	89	72
100	68	62	63
100	118	117	65
104	97	92	79
105	109	76	84
106	120	100	67
111	112	84	70
148	138	138	132

That was what Ben found when he took over the school—or at least as soon after as he was able to apply the tests.

It will be seen that not a single boy was " up to standard " in all three subjects tested, and half of them were " below standard " in every subject—even when we compare their attainments not with their real age, but with their Mental Age ! Eighteen of them were two or more years behind in one or more subjects, ten of them were three or more years behind, and of these there were some with as much as five years' retardation. One boy, for example, was eleven and a half years' old, had the *capacity* of a ten-years-old, and the *attainments* of a six-years-old.

I am not going to adduce any general argument from these particular few figures. But from all concerned with the treatment of difficult children I hear the same cry—" How *backward* they are in school ! " Dr. Cyril Burt says " Of my delinquent cases, nine out of every ten fall below the middle line of average educational attainment ; and three out of every five are so far below it as to be classifiable as technically ' backward ' in school work," and adds in a footnote that backwardness among the whole school population of London may be taken at 10 per cent.*

* " The Young Delinquent " (1927), page 336. But it is interesting to note that Healy & Bronner found only 20 per cent. retarded. ("New Light on Delinquency," p. 61).

My experience at Barns has led me to wonder whether those of us who have concentrated on the emotional causes of delinquency have not perhaps under-rated the importance of this educational factor. It is true, of course, that in very many cases the educational retardation may be a symptom having its original cause in those same emotional upsets that are also the cause of the symptoms we call delinquency. But I think there is good reason to suppose that it may sometimes be of itself a cause of behaviour problems, and certainly it greatly aggravates the behaviour difficulties.

In any case, it is certainly a problem to be tackled, and it seems to me that in any institution dealing with difficult children there should be at least one person on the teaching staff who has special qualifications in educational therapy.

Returning, however, to Ben and his problem ; it was obviously impossible, even approximately, to divide the school into classes according to age, and Ben did not attempt to do so. They were divided into two groups (as we had two teachers), the less advanced and the more advanced. Such is the heterodox nature of our school that the head teacher looks after the less advanced, for the obvious reason that the less advanced are the more difficult to teach. Even so, they are not two classes. There are about a dozen or more " classes," with only two teachers. In effect, every boy had to be treated as a separate problem though sometimes there were two or three boys who could be given the same work and could be expected to make about the same amount of progress. Ben and his colleague (Gordon T. Stubbs, Mus.Bac.) now knew, then, the degree of each boy's backwardness, and from our knowledge of their background, from our observation of them since they arrived at Barns, from diagnostic and other tests applied, they also knew pretty well the cause of the backwardness in each case. And with this knowledge, they started on their task of re-education—for that was what it amounted to in many cases.

This is not an educational treatise, and I am ignorant of the science of pedagogics. I cannot, therefore, pretend to deal with this aspect of the work in any detail—I can only give a general idea of what goes on. It was obvious above all that the first thing was to arouse and maintain each boy's interest, and this is especially so in reading and spelling. It usually happens that an older boy who cannot read has come to hate the idea of reading. One must stimulate his interest by using topics connected with his hobbies and special interests. (Richard Smith made sudden and rapid progress when he became a " Minister," and had to submit a weekly written

report to the General Meeting). Backwardness may often demand a
fresh start from the beginning, but there could be no greater mistake
than going back to infantile material. A start can be made by
building up a vocabulary of words connected with, *e.g.*, the child's
hobby. The words may be put in a book with, so far as possible,
illustrations. Pictures and word matching exercises are helpful in
securing the new knowledge. The child thus builds up his own reading
book. He knows all the words in it and will take a pride and a pleasure in reading it. The possession of this new knowledge helps to
establish confidence in himself—reading is not so far beyond his capacities after all. Another useful little dodge of Ben's (how far it is in
general use I do not know) is that, in the " wee yins' " room, every
single object has a large label tied on it bearing the name of the article,
so that by degrees the name of the object becomes as familiar as the
object itself. Many little dodges of this kind are used and they all have
as their aim the stimulation of interest, and when that is aroused
the individual difficulties that the tests have shewn, can be dealt
with.

In all cases it is important that the child should play an active
part in the process of learning, and he must be provided with
materials that make this possible. Materials of this nature have been
issued by educational publishers, but it is a good thing for a teacher
to make his own materials to meet his own needs—or get the children
to make them ! There are masses of reading books for children at the
infant level—but they are intended for infants, not boys of ten and
eleven ! And they all have the major drawback of being in print
instead of cursive writing, which is apt to add to the confusion.
It is found to be an enormous advantage not to teach reading
letter by letter, but by whole words, each word being conceived
as a unity in itself, and not a number of little bits. Cursive writing
adds to this conception as script detracts from it. This method has
the advantage of making use of kinesthetic memory—the child
is able to remember not only what the word looks like when it is
written, but what it *feels* like when you write it ; the feeling then is
about the whole word, and not about odd letters. This is of
particular value in teaching left-lateral pupils (of whom we have
so many) who may be able to write on to the end of the word when
once they start it, provided they conceive it as one design. If,
however, they think of it as several little designs in a row, they are
very likely indeed to get the order confused. Most of the remedial
exercises in reading and spelling have, therefore, been prepared by
hand. Use has been made of graded word-and-picture-matching
schemes, together with appropriate phonic lists, sentence building,

individual picture dictionaries, wall dictionaries, and so forth. Ben's inventiveness is as endless as his enthusiasm.

In arithmetic, too, it was found necessary to prepare pupil-teacher cards to meet individual needs. Professor Schonell's method of learning multiplication and division facts is used extensively.*

Throughout the whole field of remedial work it was found that the first element of success lay in the simple fact that the child's difficulties had been recognised ; that they were a cause for sympathetic concern and not for blame ; and that they were receiving individual attention. If the child receives sympathy and encouragement, and if there is regular progress and systematic revision, he soon begins to feel that he is getting somewhere, and will happily accept really hard work. Hence the cheers referred to in Chapter One, when " extra school " was announced.

I have often regretted, when I have been speaking or writing about our work, that there is no way of weighing or measuring the progress made by a boy in the overcoming of those difficulties for which he is referred to us. One can *see* changes, and often remarkable changes. One can see a sullen, furtive, frightened child develop into a bright, open, happy person. But what a help it would be in our publicity if we could express that progress in figures ! We have to manage as well as we can without, but in this particular aspect of our work we *can* give figures, and I beg leave to remind the reader that the methods that have produced these figures are the same methods, in principle, as those which produce, the other, imponderable results. But as they have been applied to the other, outside-school, part of the work longer than they have been applied in the school, the presumption is that the results in that field are even more gratifying.

All that as a prologue to the statistics given below. When Ben had been at work a year, he applied the attainments tests again to see whether progress was being made. I give below the figures which were produced for the 20 boys who took both lots of tests.

There are nine boys fewer here than on the list shewn on page 115 ; this is merely because nine boys left during the year in question. The last boy on the list with his I.Q. of 148, is quite obviously out of his element in our school, and as soon as his behaviour difficulties shewed signs of clearing up he was sent to the High School.

These figures, if you will be good enough to give them the attention

* F. J. Schonell—" Backwardness in the Basic Subjects."

Attainments Quotients in :—

Intelligence Quotients	READING			SPELLING			ARITHMETIC*		
	First Test	Second Test	Progress in months	First Test	Second Test	Progress in months	First Test	Second Test	Progress in months
72	78	77	7	65	66	8	90	88	4
75	79	86	19	70	72	12	73	87	28
77	64	73	24	59	55	3	61	63	8
78	56	67	20	58	63	12	58	70	19
78	111	113	16	102	100	10	90	92	7
78	70	?	?	66	66	8	74	81	16
85	81	86	16	80	75	5	88	103	24
85	55	61	17	50	58	18	74	86	24
86	60	76	29	60	71	22	Infant level		
88	105	103	8	97	95	9	76	78	8
89	90	93	20	77	73	7	49	64	9
89	78	87	22	71	75	12	58	60	9
97	92	102	22	80	72	6	63	68	9
97	124	127	17	102	104	15	77	79	7
100	68	81	23	62	63	12	63	73	17
100	118	116	12	117	100	6	65	70	15
104	97	114	32	92	94	15	79	96	19
105	109	116	21	76	89	26	84	80	3
111	112	110	8	84	92	19	70	71	6
148	138	127	?	138	106	?	132	130	?

* The Arithmetic results are after a *six* and not a twelve month interval.

they deserve, speak for themselves, and should be enough to silence any doubter. Not every boy made astonishing progress during the year, there are still some whose difficulties are not properly understood ; especially in spelling, but they will be dealt with in time. One of the objects of the test was to find out how many of the boys were being successfully dealt with, and further investigations will now be needed in the case of those who have not made satisfactory progress. But in the main, the picture is one of most extraordinary progress, and one such as any teacher might be very proud of. It must be borne in mind, too, that there has been no cramming or anything like it. Barns boys go to school for an hour a day less than most State schoolboys, and this progress is all the result of happy, purposeful work, which has given pleasure to the boys in the same degree as their results have given satisfaction to the teachers.

I end this chapter with a few lines from Ben's report to the Committee when these results of his first year's work were known :—

" There have been occasions when I have felt that we stressed freedom and self-discipline to the detriment of quietness and dignity, and in using individual self-activity methods, we ran the risk of losing the steady progress which more formal teaching was designed to secure. It is very gratifying to discover that the way we have always felt to be right has now been proved to be so."

CHAPTER TWELVE

PRUDES AND BESOMS*

"Who said, Ay, mum's the word'?"
WALTER DE LA MARE—"The Song of the Mad Prince."

I COMPLAINED in Chapter Two about a certain lack of moral sense among Barns boys. That was true, so far as it went. Particularly in relation to questions of *meum* and *tuum* and similar aspects of social life does their behaviour seem to be based more on fear of consequences than upon any opinion as to the rightness or wrongness of a particular piece of behaviour. But in the sphere of the emotions—on questions of their feelings about people—they are apt to acquire enormous and overburdening feelings of guilt, to which I have referred elsewhere. These guilt feelings are not necessarily conscious—rather the contrary—though in a young child they are not buried so deep in the unconscious as they are likely to be in the case of an adult. But there is one type of behaviour which is almost invariably felt to be wicked beyond measure—though not necessarily therefore to be avoided ! I refer to the type of behaviour which they describe as " dirty."

I suspect that this conscious feeling of guilt about " dirty " things is even more pronounced among Scottish children than among their English equivalents. My friend Reginald Reynolds, in his admirable book " Cleanliness and Godliness," complains about the debasement of the English language so that it is no longer polite to refer to a water closet, which has therefore, come to be known as a place for washing oneself. But the word lavatory itself is now hardly decent, and he wonders how long it will be before the word bathroom brings a blush to the cheek of the modest. In some parts of Scotland at least, that day is very near. Among the boys who come to Barns, " bathroom " does not in the least, mean what it means to you and me. It is associated in their minds purely and simply (if such an association can be either pure or simple) with its secondary function, and they are genuinely surprised when you explain to them what its primary function is. They think you are trying to be funny and in some vague way, dirty—just as a cockney

---

* " Bisms ! " Barns boys pronounce it, and they mean something of a minx and something of a trollope.

child might if you were to tell him that a lavatory is a place for washing. Not only is a privy which contains nothing but a close-stool, invariably known as a bathroom, the acts of micturition and defæcation are called " doing a bathroom."

This excessive delicacy is not confined to matters of bodily evacuation. It applies to the whole body, and it applies beyond everything else to matters of sex.

Nor is it the child of ignorance. There are very few boys who come to Barns—at however early an age—without some kind of working knowledge of the "facts of life." I well remember one day during our first winter, walking along the drive with Sammy Johnson. He was chatting away as we walked, and I have to confess that I was taking very little notice of what he was saying. Sammy was very backward (he was not yet nine), his speech was babyish and his diction was very bad, so listening was rather a strain when one considers that there was also the Edinburgh accent (with which I was not as yet very familiar) to cope with. Presently however, hearing Jean's name mentioned several times, I pricked up my ears and began to pay attention. He was not really talking to me. He was " fantasying " aloud, and his fantasy was, if you please, an elaborate fantasy of sexual intercourse !

Copulation is, to many of our boys, a commonplace idea before they come to us, but the odd thing is that it is none the less regarded as a disgustingly dirty practice ! This attitude they must have acquired either from their parents or from other boys in their environment who had got it from *their* parents.

Among what are sometimes known as " the lower orders " sexual intercourse begins too often in a furtive, sniggering, groping manipulation of each other's genitalia in dark doorways, in " the pictures," or on a park bench, until marriage provides them with a bed, a licence for further intimacy (if indeed the marriage is not the result of further intimacy) and public approval of the inevitable result. There is no doubt that this nasty, furtive, sniggering attitude is carried over into the intercourse of ordinary married life. In far too many cases, in poor and overcrowded districts, children sleep in the same room as their parents until a late age. They have listened at night to sniggerings and furtive mutterings coming from the other bed, carried out in the particular tone of voice which is associated with " dirty " things. They have heard all these things and, very naturally, they have investigated. When their investigations take the form of direct questions they are often told, either sniggeringly or indignantly, not to be " dirty ", and it is made quite clear that the whole thing is something the adults are ashamed of. It soon becomes obvious to the child that something " dirty " is going on, and it is not very long before he finds out what that " dirty " thing is.

Miss Melanie Klein, the eminent psychoanalyst of children, appears to trace a large number of child-neuroses with which she dealt, to the fact of the child having witnessed what she calls "the primal scene."[*] Not for one moment would I like to be thought that I dispute her findings—even if I were qualified to do so. But most of the children she treated seem to have been middle-class children, brought up to " middle-class morality," to whom witnessing the primal scene would be most unusual and exceptional, and hence tend to be traumatic. Some of our children have been more frequent witnesses of the primal scene, and while I do not deny that it may in some cases lead to neurosis, and while it may be an important cause of their difficulties, what it does undoubtedly lead to is a sordid and nasty conception of the relation of the sexes, and a state of unhappy and complete bewilderment that their own parents should be habitually " dirty," and above all, that life itself is the result of behaviour they are brought up to regard as " dirty." What a puzzling and difficult world ! After all, if my parents are dirty, why shouldn't I be dirty ? For they are not told that these things, like smoking and drinking and staying up late, are the preserve of adulthood, but merely that they are dirty.[†]

We have to try at Barns to cope with this situation. We cannot do it as well as I should like, and I have come at length to the conclusion that we cannot hope to do it unless we have girls as well as boys in the hostel. The superficial " progressive " may think that this should have been obvious all along, and that we should have been co-educational from the start. It is not as simple as all that. In the first place, co-education must not be confused with co-re-education, if I may make that ugly word even uglier—and our work is both. To take children of both sexes from respectable homes at an early age and educate them together is one thing, and perhaps a good thing. But the re-education together of boys and girls with this unhealthy attitude to and precocious knowledge of sexual matters, is something that needs to be thought over at least twice before it is plunged into. Then it appears that there are far more " difficult " boys than girls and we should probably have had great difficulty in keeping something like an even balance of the sexes. There was the fact, too, in our case that the house available

---

[*] The Psychoanalysis of Children.

[†] I should not like it to be thought that I believe this nasty, sniggering attitude to sex to be confined to the " lower orders.". I know, alas, that it is not. But among them it is more easily and more early transmitted to the children than among " respectable " families.

to us was not well suited to the accommodation of both sexes. Further, while our work is experimental, it would have been unwise to experiment in too many fields at once. Finally, I myself, have had very little experience with girls, and none with difficult girls. So, taking all these factors into consideration it was decided— and I think in all the circumstances, rightly decided—to take only boys. I think, though, that if there is a next time for me, I shall be, on the whole, against segregation, in spite of my own inexperience.

Before I came to Scotland I was for a short time in charge of a hostel for somewhat similar children in the South. We found there that some of the boys were friendly with some girls in the village. They seemed to regard this as something they must be surreptitious about, so we tried to bring it into the open. We had a birthday party and invited all the girls. As the evening wore on we noticed that the girls seemed to need to " leave the room " a very large number of times, and presently we discovered that every time they went in to a W.C. they took a boy in with them. These girls really were "dirty " and I, who have perhaps seen more than the average of what sentimental writers call " the sordid side of life," was shocked at what I discovered about their conversation and conduct. Eventually (though not until my wife had tried running a club for them) we had to exclude them from the hostel. I am not among those who are horrified at the idea of children inspecting and experimenting with one another. But I confess that I am horrified by the idea of a boy's only contact with girls being of a kind which he considers dirty. For there is such a thing as dirt in sex, even if, like beauty, it is in the eye of the beholder.

We had a similar experience at Barns. Some of the older boys became " pally " with some girls from the town. I did not imagine that we should have a second time, the experience we had suffered before. But we did. Once again I encouraged them to come up to the Hostel, and once again they were unusually unpleasant little creatures whose aim in making the acquaintance of the boys was solely to display themselves and swop dirty stories. If those girls had been resident at Barns it would not have mattered. There would then have been ample opportunity for every kind of healthy relationship with the boys, in addition to the sexual investigatory relationship, which we should soon have been able to put on a healthy basis. But since it seemed that their only contact was to be a sniggering one, I discouraged it.

This was the beginning of what later blossomed into my weekly "hygiene " class. I am not a teacher, but I have usually helped out with the teaching in a minor way. At this time I used to have a group of the older boys in my sitting-room for poetry. The boys happened to be mostly the ones who had been entangled with the nasty little girls, so I thought I would try to explain my attitude. We, therefore, scrapped poetry for a few weeks in favour of sex talks. First we had a few talks on the machinery of reproduction, to make sure they had the facts right. I was able to tell them very little they didn't know, except a few technical terms which they then bandied about with great pride. A few were glad to have their minds set at rest about the naturalness and innocence of morning erections which they had just begun to experience, and there were gaps here and there which I was able to fill in. But by and large, they were pretty well informed. Indeed, in the four years we have been here, I only recall one case of gross anatomical misinformation, and that appears to have been somewhat obsessional in nature.

I then tried to explain how it was that while sex is not itself " dirty," it could be made so by people having a nasty attitude to it. It is a difficult idea to put across to boys of 11, 12 and 13, and how much success I had I do not know. But I think something reached them.

A little while after this Ben asked me to take a weekly " Hygiene " Class, which I have been doing ever since. This " Hygiene " is a mixture of Anatomy, Biology, Physiology and Sexology, and it goes down very well. I am an authority on none of these subjects, and my method is the time-honoured one of keeping one jump ahead of the class. It includes such things as, on the one hand, the structure of the body, and on the other the reason for keeping the nose clean ; how the muscles work (and I find I am not the only one who doesn't understand this) and why bowels must be opened regularly ; what happens to your food when you've swallowed it, and where babies come from. Everything that can have anything to do with the body is dragged in (so far as I can find out anything about it !) and things hitherto regarded as " dirty " are put (I hope !) in their proper place. For, however much faulty information I may impart on subjects which, I am astonished to find, are still little understood by the experts, I believe we really are getting sex out of the realm of dirt and sniggering and furtiveness.

The house is on the banks of the Tweed, so there is a great deal of bathing, which is all (so far as the boys are concerned) done in the innocent nude, and it has come to be accepted as a perfectly natural thing. So much so, that when we went to camp they all jumped into the farmer's duck-pond in the same natural way, and were indignantly chased out by the farmer as a set of " dirty little rascals." I had carefully brought along some bathing slips (improvised) against this contingency, but they just couldn't be bothered with them, and the voluntary helper who was supervising the bathing was not experienced enough in the ways of the world to guess what a Border farmer's attitude to nudity was likely to be ! Very often, when signs of puberty begin to show themselves a boy is reluctant to go in if the womenfolk are about, but I see nothing unhealthy in a certain measure of modesty in the adolescent.

For the rest, sex re-education takes place all day and every day. By maintaining a healthy attitude ourselves, and by encouraging them to talk openly and naturally of things they had hitherto considered dirty, we hope that we are gradually fostering a healthy attitude in the boys. But although it may be healthier when they leave than when they come, we can do little about helping them to get along easily and naturally with girls, until we have some girls living in the family.

It will be noticed that I have said nothing about masturbation. If this is a problem at Barns, I am blind to it. It is true that in the early days, before our efforts at sex-education had got under way, one or two of the older boys, I heard, were worried about masturbation—but not, I believe, seriously. It must be remembered that boys of the Barns type have not been subjected to " middle-class morality," and therefore, do not seem to have been told any of the perfectly ridiculous and dreadful things that are often told to boys a little higher up in the social scale about bodily decay and mental derangement following this common practice. These boys of whom I spoke were just a little worried because, as what they had been doing was connected with parts of their anatomy they considered dirty, then their behaviour was dirty and they were a little worried about it. I tried, with how much success I do not know, to set their minds at rest. But among the boys who have been growing up at Barns since then, there is in the main, an attitude to sex sufficiently healthy to prevent masturbation becoming the problem it is with some boys. The principal damage done by masturbation is caused by undue worrying about it. The fact of worrying about it keeps it constantly in the mind, giving it a somewhat obsessive quality, thus increasing its frequency, hence greater worry—and so on. This is a thing about which it is very easy to be misunderstood, and I should not like it to be thought that my attitude is merely one of " Oh, masturbation, that's nothing—don't worry about *that*." It is an undesirable practice, however common it may be, but its evils have been in the past grossly exaggerated, and it seems to me that it is better to treat it as an undesirable, but not a frightfully sinful or harmful practice, which one should try to overcome, like nail-biting and similar practices. And I do think that it is perhaps better for a boy to worry too little about it than to worry too much. However that may be, sex among Barns boys—at least when they have been with us a year or two—is not something to worry about, so masturbation is not a problem among them.

I know that to the psychoanalyst the latency period (during which most of our boys come to us) is a period of intense conflict about masturbation. But it is an unconscious conflict. I know too, that the psychoanalyst would say that during the latency period two things are essential if the boy is to develop normally. He must be sure of the love and approval of his " objects " (usually the parents or parent substitutes) and he must be given a sense of achievement. Perhaps it is because at Barns we concentrate on these two things that the boys seem to emerge from latency into adolescence with no serious masturbation problem.

CHAPTER THIRTEEN

THE SONS OF THE FATHERS

" . . . in like way is all hidden when we would backward see from what regì
of remoteness the whatness of our whoness hath fetched his whenceness."
JAMES JOYCE—" Ulysses."

I SAID I should probably refer again to the story of Stephen Baillie.
I cannot give as many details of the family as I should like, as
obviously, I cannot run the risk of its being recognised. Baillie
senior was, according to several social work agencies which had
dealings with the family, a difficult, aggressive, self-opinionated
man, completely dominating his wife, who seemed an inoffensive
little woman, perhaps indulgent to her children, and very easily
swayed by them or by him. They had a medium-sized family,
one member of which was in an Approved School. They dis-
claimed strongly that they had any difficulty with Stevie, but the
mother gladly accepted the suggestion that he should be evacuated
to Barns. He had been truanting, staying out late and going with a
rough gang of boys, although he was only nine, and there seems
also to have been a certain amount of pilfering. . He had been
evacuated once before, but returned as incorrigible. The father
was not so keen on the idea of Stevie's evacuation, but gave in to
Stevie's pleading, which was the more urgent because his mother
had assured him that among the attractions of Barns was the fact
that there was " nae schule." She afterwards admitted the lie
quite unashamedly, saying she thought it would encourage him to
go to Barns.

Stevie arrived then in July, 1940. He came with another little
boy of about the same age whom he promptly claimed (though
without the slightest foundation) as a cousin, and over whom he
early established an ascendancy which seems to have been modelled
on his father's relation to his mother. Wee Sandy Sporran and he
were almost inseparable for some weeks, though always " charging "
one another. It soon began to be apparent that Stevie was using
Sandy to do his dirty work for him—Sandy did the pilfering and
Stevie took the profits. However, there was no occasion for us to
take any action about that because as soon as Sandy began to find
his way around he started charging Stevie for his various assaults
upon his integrity, and after a while the partnership was broken.

But his capacity to dominate other boys remained a characteristic of Stevie all the time he was with us. It was not done by bullying or any kind of terrorisation—he had not the physique for that. It was done by charm of manner, persuasiveness and a glib tongue. Though a noisy, strident, mischievous little boy (he once laid a trail of tin-tacks on the stairs down which the boys go, barefoot, to their bath) he could, if he wanted to ingratiate himself, switch on a most soulful expression in his beautiful big eyes with their long lashes. He seemed to find it more easy to lie than not. When asked a question a lie sprang to his lips (it seemed) as spontaneously as the truth to anyone else's, and if he paused before replying it was probably because he was going to speak the truth. He always had a reply ready, and was strong in defence of his rights—one who could develop into an excellent example of what is known as a " lag's lawyer."

We described him during his first few weeks as " An incorrigible thief and liar . . . Loves screaming, and will make himself so difficult at bedtime that he sometimes has to be forcibly undressed, during which time he screams continuously." (This note makes me smile. The idea of Jean, who was in charge of him at that time, " forcibly " undressing anyone is a little quaint. But I suppose that would be what she called it.) ". . . Spits in people's faces . . . language to Jean deplorable . . . very high-spirited . . . in some ways the most spirited boy here . . . " By December—a mere five months later—we were able to note, " A happy purposeful child now, presenting no serious problem but gains need to be consolidated." The reason we noted that gains needed to be consolidated was that, although lying and stealing and screaming and spitting were gone, he still displayed a much milder symptom of insecurity—he was never happy unless he had a " keeper." That is to say, he was continually committing offences not serious in themselves, but which might involve us in trouble with our neighbours—trespassing in game woods, and that sort of thing. The reply of the Committee to such offences is usually a restriction of freedom as a preventive measure. At first the restriction is a mild one, but if that does not answer the restriction becomes more and more severe until at last the boy concerned may be handed over to the care of a " keeper," with whom he has to stay at all times, and who is responsible for keeping him out of mischief. This sounds like a very severe sentence but actually it is rarely anything of the sort. Very often the offender will contrive to be given as keeper, someone whom he likes and the two become real companions so that the conditions of their partnership are irksome to neither. It will readily be seen that this is admirable " medicine " for a boy who is beginning to feel less insecure but has not quite found his feet yet, and Stevie for some months absolutely insisted on having a keeper. Whenever the keeper was " taken off," he soon saw to it that one was " put on " again. Stevie then was going steadily forward. But three months later—in March, 1941— we find this note :—" Very serious lapse since last note. Fractious, stealing, tremendous amount of hoarding, which seems chief pre-occupation, especially of stolen goods. Seems to have stolen £1 from D.W., 10/- from G.T. (two visitors), 2/- from office in copper and several other sums, besides cutlery, etc.—all for hoarding " in various " hidey-holes " about the place. (It will be recalled that some of the more serious thefts had not been committed by Stevie at all—he had merely directed suspicion to himself ; but this had not become clear at the time the note was made (*see page* 19). " Now having weekly talks with Wills, from which it appears that father recently died—apparently about time of relapse. But stories of father's death vary, and it may be pure fantasy. Wills to have enquiries made." Well—we had enquiries made. Stevie said his information had come from his mother, so our enquiries began with her. She was very vague about it all, but " didn't think " she had told Stevie his father was dead. She said her husband was away on Government work, but admitted that she had not heard from him for some months and that he was not supporting her. " From information received," however (to use that very useful police formula) it soon became clear to us that Baillie had deserted, and when there was no further doubt about this I sought an interview with Stephen. I told him his father was not dead. To my suggestion that he already knew this, his reply was indeterminate. Then I told him quite bluntly that, in fact, his father had deserted. His reaction astonished me and confirmed my impression that he had known all along. Without pausing for thought or for question or for further elucidation, he burst forth into a torrent of the most foul, obscene and offensive vituperative against his father (with a few by-blows at me). That finished me with Stevie. He had thought a good deal of his father, and I, as father surrogate, had enjoyed the advantage of that. Refusing to believe ill of him, he had " killed him "—or he had " killed " him for refusing to live up to the standard Stevie had set for him ; or of course—which is more likely—he killed him for an illogical amalgam of both these reasons. Now I had insisted on bringing him to life again, and had substituted for the dead hero, a living rogue. Very good ; I was still father surrogate, and there were no more weekly talks with me.

But from that moment we began to see an improvement in

I

Stevie again. He did not change overnight, but having accepted the facts, he began to adjust himself to them. He began, slowly, to be less interested in hoarding (and stealing things to hoard), there was less talk about hidey-holes, less lying and—most interesting of all, he restored his father to us. He had given various staff members at various times, accounts of his father's demise. Now to each of them he gave, at odd times, equally imaginary accounts of his father's present activities, differing in many particulars, but all agreeing in the one particular that his pursuits were now mundane and not celestial. I see, on looking back at the notes we made about that time, that we attempted what I described as a " tentative interpretation." " Mother told him father had deserted," though perhaps not in so many words. He therefore " killed " father in fantasy and thus (a) wants to bury him to get him out of his mind (hiding and hoarding) ; (b) wants to be punished for his crime (" naughty " behaviour, directing suspicion to himself, etc.) and (c) feels insecure owing to loss of father and wants to hedge himself about with lies, etc. (a form of hiding and protection). Doubtless, too, the knowledge of various articles hidden in places known only to him would tend to make him feel less insecure. Whether this makes sense or not Stevie slowly got better and better as we did our best to provide him with security on a deeper level than lies and hidey-holes, so that by the following spring, he had marched steadily forward to the state he had been in before his relapse. An interesting contributory factor in his recovery, as well as a measure of its progress, was an ingenious idea of Jean's. She gave him a " bank " containing several coins. This he treasured very highly, going to bed every night with it under his pillow for some weeks. When he began to feel a littler happier he manœuvred the coins out of the box and spent them, but still kept the box religiously under his pillow like a talisman. After a few more weeks, however, even that became unnecessary, and Stevie was his own man again. Ben told us that in school, during the " relapsed " period, Steven had been most reluctant to do any new work, but as he began to mend he was " now more ready to tackle new things and works away steadily (January, 1942)." By the summer of 1942 we had ceased to worry about Master Baillie, and were merely watching, with some satisfaction if not even complacency, the slow consolidation of gains made. Alas, there was little time for consolidation. In July his mother took him away. I did my best to prevent her, but it seemed that her husband was back again and had decided to have Stevie home. His conscience was at work, I imagine. Poor Stevie thought he was going home for a holiday, and was annoyed when, on reaching home, he found he was expected to stay. He soon began badgering his parents to allow him to come back to Barns, but it was not until he had been home seven months that he was successful. He returned to Barns in February, 1943, his mother having given a solemn undertaking that there was to be no more snatching away.

He was not the same as the Stevie that left. There was a hard look in his eye (for of course he was " back " again in more senses than one), was more calculating in his lies, and more difficult to detect. Instead of stealing fairly light-heartedly, he planned ahead, invariably implicating someone else, and generally seeing to it that they got the blame. We saw that we had to start all over again, and that it was likely to be as difficult a job as ever.

As soon as he arrived, he wanted to go home again. We are always reluctant to take back boys who have been left some time, because while in the drab surroundings of their homes they form a highly idealised picture of Barns in their minds, and the reality is apt to be a disappointment. We made an exception in Stevie's case because—well, because he was Stevie I suppose ! Well, we got over that stile, and it was not many days before he had stopped talking about going home again. But beyond that, progress was very, very slow, and when he had been back three months I upset everything. I shouted at him. In all conscience I had cause enough, though I will not weary you with that, and few people would have contented themselves with merely shouting. But it was a mistake. He told his father. He did not improve on the occasion, as boys often do when they are feeling disgruntled, by saying I had beaten him or thrown him about. He told his father simply that I had shouted at him, and that was enough—his father came for him. In reply to my reasonings, my implorings, my begging and praying, my coaxing and wheedling, Mr. Baillie favoured me with a short lecture on the proper way to deal with sensitive children who should, I was told, never be shouted at— having five minutes earlier told me that Stevie would be well chastised if he tried his monkey tricks at home ! I reminded him of the definite undertaking Mrs. Baillie had given me that Stevie was to stay here this time. He simply laughed at that. And finally, when I saw that it really was quite impossible to keep Stevie (for it would be useless to have him back again, supposing his parents were willing after a few more months), feeling that I was entitled to some little recompense, I gave myself the supreme pleasure of telling Baillie Senior what I thought about him, in simple but not, I fear, in dignified English. You may think that such a course would do no one any good. It did me a great deal of good, and I fear that the unsuspecting

I*

Mr. Baillie got a good deal of what I had often longed to say to many parents.

This long story is not strictly a true one. It is merely founded on fact, and I have altered it in several material particulars so that none may say " That is I " or " that is he." But I have altered it in no way that affects the validity of the moral I wish to draw. That moral is, simply, that people like my " Baillies " are not fit to have the custody of children, and should have their children taken from them. As the law stands to-day, that cannot be done, or it cannot be done without a great deal of difficulty. The law does, of course, allow of the removal of children from the custody of their parents. Broadly speaking, it may be done if the children are being grossly neglected or cruelly ill-treated physically or if they are being subjected to immoral influences. Unfortunately, immoral in this context always seems to refer to sexual immorality such as living in a brothel or being the subjects of incest. If I were to go to court and say " Tom Jones is being subjected to immoral influence. Both his parents are liars," I'm afraid it is very unlikely that any serious action would be taken.

It is true also that a child who has committed a crime may be removed from his parents' control by committal to a " fit person " who is to all intents and purposes *in loco parentis*. But the trouble with this is that the child must commit an offence before it happens, and in any case it is not used (in my opinion) half often enough, owing to the sentimental prejudice that exists against taking children from their homes. I have nothing against the home as an institution. I merely claim that many boys of the kind I am concerned with haven't got a home in any real sense, and in acting in the way I suggest you are not depriving him of a home, you are giving him one—often for the first time in his life. " A bad home," say the ignorant sentimentalists " is better than none." I do not know exactly what they mean by a bad home, but I am certain that a good foster-home, second best though it be, is immeasurably better than the sort of place so many boys of the Barns type are brought up in.

Stevie Baillie is a good example of the sort of thing I mean, but please do not for one moment imagine that—among Barns boys and their kind—he is by any means an isolated case. " Is your mother," I said hesitatingly, to Cecil Bryant, " always strictly truthful ? " " I dinny ken," he said, " I think she is when she's talking to other grown-ups ; but she isna wi' us." That was a large part of the trouble with Cecil and his brother, Harry. His mother 'phoned one day from a call-box—would we send the boys home for a short holiday next morning ? As it was in the school holidays we complied without question. When they got home there was no mother there —she had disappeared and no-one knew where she was, so they were packed off to Barns by Grannie. A few weeks later she was promising to come and see them " next visiting Sunday," but nothing ever came of it. Then they were to go home for a holiday at Christmas. " I'll come and fetch you next Wednesday," said the letter, but there was no sign of mother on Wednesday.' " Coming for you Saturday," said the wire, but no sign of mother on Saturday. Then there was silence until the middle of the term, when a letter came—for me this time—saying she was coming for the boys " on Sunday " and giving various reasons why I should let them home during mid-term, for a whole fortnight. The letter came on Saturday, so that was no time to reply. She followed it the same afternoon. If I had tried to insist that the boys were not to go home in mid-term we might have lost them altogether, so I let them go. They were away three weeks, and returned without overcoats or ration books, but with—in the case of Cecil anyway—a very nasty temper. Like so many mothers, she tried to atone for months of neglect by a few weeks of over-indulgence. They went to the pictures every day for three weeks, and when the time came for them to return to Barns they were told " I'll be having you home for good in the summer."

Before this Cecil had been making great strides, in spite of the many unkept promises. Stealing had completely stopped, tantrums were rare, he was making a real contribution to the general well-being and was working hard for his " qualifying exam." He was eager and purposeful, and we were proud of him. After his three weeks at home he just flopped. No stealing, it is true, but foul temper, listlessness, carelessness and no interest in anything. Why ? Partly because mother said he was " going home for good " before long, which itself would be unsettling enough, but partly also, and this is a large part, because *he didn't know whether to believe her or not.* You who have been brought up in respectable and well-conducted homes where the only lie that is known is the social taradiddle, imagine what it must be like to have a mother whom you know to be a liar, and whose word you can never trust. How can such a child feel stable and secure ? Is there any reason under the sun why a woman like this, simply because of the biological accident of being their physical mother, should be allowed and, indeed, encouraged, to play fast and loose with the lives of human beings ?

Then there was Mrs. Goff. Dan Goff came to us because he was a persistent truant, a shocking liar, and quite beyond his parents' control. His father was a deserter in the military as well as in the matrimonial sense. Mrs. Goff used to send letters to Daniel in which

she discussed the sexual aberrations of her husband and her friends
with the utmost candour—Daniel then being 10 years old. When I
discovered that I took to censoring Dan's incoming mail, much to
the annoyance of the mother. Then father, having been recovered
by the military and having consequently served a spell in gaol,
thought he might as well return also to matrimony, took control
of the family and ordered Daniel's return home. Before Dan had
been home three months he appeared in the Court on his mother's
prosecution, as being " beyond parents' control." The charge
was dropped on it being agreed that Daniel should return to Barns.
What they had been doing to him I do not know, but he was so
terrified as he got near to Barns that I did not re-introduce him to
his friends at first, but put him straight to bed in the sick-room
so that he could find his feet gradually. From the sick-room,
before he had so much as seen another boy, he wrote to his mother
saying how he was being bullied by the other boys here. At least
he wrote a letter. Before it was time to post it he was feeling a
little better, so it didn't go. That by the way. From that moment
until the present time, 18 months later, the mother has not sent him
a single letter that has not been concerned with some plan to get
Daniel back home again, by subterfuge or downright deceit.
On one occasion she begged him home " for one day " for his
sister's birthday. I could not resist this, because Daniel was so
keen on it. He had had a letter once before (which somehow
evaded my censorship) in which his mother had told him to " come
home for good," sending him the fare, but he had decided—of
his own free will—that he was better off at Barns. Another time
when his mother wanted him home for a holiday he had cheerfully
agreed with me that once he got home he would probably stay there,
so he'd better not go. So I felt that there was a good chance of his
being able to resist his mother's blandishments, though that in
itself would not have been sufficient reason for my agreeing to his
going home if there had not been the additional reason that Daniel
had made some very nice toys for his sister at woodwork, and it
seemed a pity not to let him have the pleasure of giving them to
her. So he went—for one day. He came back, seven weeks later,
after much pressure from me, from Hilda Ludlam (our social worker)
and from the School Attendance Officer. I afterwards learned
that he had been working on a milk round all this time—during
school hours, too. In a way I was glad of this, because it enabled me,
the last time Mrs. Goff tried to get Daniel away, to threaten her
with prosecution, which at any rate has silenced her for a few
weeks. Relations between Mrs. Goff and us are, therefore, rather

bad, but the extraordinary thing is that from the very moment Daniel came here—quite voluntarily, and at his parents' request —she has insisted on treating us as enemies of her and of her boy. Hilda Ludlam has never had from her anything but abuse, and I— though I have never seen her—am never referred to but with oaths and obscenity.

In what sense is it right to leave any child in such hands?

Not, let me hasten to add, that it is always the mother that is to blame. Mrs. Johnson is pretty harmless, though weak and vacillating. Her husband is a little, drunken, violent tough. By some amazing Mendelian freak they have bred a son who is gentle, intelligent and sensitive. Not, as I almost wrote, acutely sensitive, but very surprisingly so, compared with his father. To Mr. Johnson, Paul is just " no bloody good." He has always been treated with the utmost contempt by his father and it is not surprising that this boy, who really has excellent qualities, should have an intense sense of inferiority. We have worked hard to eradicate it, and not entirely without success. But he cannot face the prospect of going to live with strangers, so when he is 14 he will go home. I tremble to think of the result. What an astonishing law it is that compels this lamb to lie down with that lion—to be accurate, which prevents us from removing this lamb from that lion's den. For there is nothing in law that we can do—at least until Paul commits a crime, and then he will probably be put on probation as a first offender, and kept at home to suffer the increased opprobrium of his father.

In considering what I should write in this chapter I compiled a list of examples I could quote. I have by no means exhausted them —indeed they could in themselves fill a book. There must be thousands of such homes. What can be done about them? Manifestly, society cannot employ an army of Paul Prys to ferret their way into all the homes in the United Kingdom to see whether parents are fit to have the custody of their children. But when the facts are discovered—as they often are—by Probation Officers, Social Workers and others, then the law should provide a remedy.

I imagine that hostels of the Barns type have come to stay. There are only two that I know of in Scotland, but I gather that there are many in England, though the powers that be do not seem anxious that they should know much about each other. They are —for the most part—at present part of the Evacuation Scheme and, of course, if they are to continue after the war some different kind of legislative provision will have to be made for them. I hope I am not too sanguine in assuming that that will be done. When it *is* done, I hope and pray there will be some means by which

Wardens or Headmasters or whatever they may be called, may be given a status—where the facts warrant it—*in loco parentis* in the legal sense, not only during the period of the child's residence in the hostel, but for some years afterwards.

In one case and one case only (and that because Peebles has an unusually enlightened Sheriff substitute) I have had a Barns boy committed to me as a "fit person" until he is 18. There is not the slightest doubt that it is this fact and, so far as I can see, only this fact, that has prevented his entering a career of crime. He is now 16 (and of course no longer resident at Barns) and although he has given us some anxious moments, all seems set fair now.

I am convinced that in a large number of cases the cure for juvenile crime is—take them out of their own homes, cut them off from their parents and give them a new, real home and new parents. Take them away not for a year or two, at an Approved School, but for good. The ideal thing in many cases is a foster home, but ,the small hostel is sometimes almost as good and often is much better.

I have in no way exaggerated the problem of inadequate or unsuitable homes and as I have said I could have given many more instances. But if I have implied that *all* the parents of Barns boys are fools or rogues or both, then I have overstated my case. True there are very few where the parental relationship is ideal, but in many cases that is due to no fault of the parents and in others it is due to the unhappy fact of love having flown out of the window.

Even where the parents are "to blame," how are we to blame them? It is easier to blame the parents than the children, because one expects adult behaviour from adults (goodness knows why!—one rarely sees it!) and because one realises that the child's background has made it almost impossible for him to be other than he is. Ian Burns's mother, though a pleasant enough woman, seemed to have no affection whatever for her children, and no control over them, and they seemed to have had no kind of moral training. They frequently had scabies and—her husband being abroad—she would leave them alone in the house while she went off to the "pictures" or to dances. On one occasion there was a fire in the house while she was out enjoying herself. Her mother-in-law (who had been strongly opposed to the marriage) had no good word to say for her, and more than once threatened to call in the N.S.P.C.C. With such a background, what do you *expect* the children to be like?

But what of *Mrs. Burns's* background. When we learn that her parents abandoned her at an early age; that she was brought up in a particularly soul-less orphanage under strict discipline and never in her life knew what it was to be loved, we shall find it difficult to condemn her if she seems unable to love her children. When we learn that the people among whom she was brought up believed that the only kind of " success " open to a girl was to secure a husband for herself as soon as possible and thus escape the disciplined drudgery by which they earned their living—when we understand that, we are not surprised that she leapt at the first chance of a husband when she was barely 17. I seem to be writing of the Victorian age—but Mrs. Burns was only in her twenties when her first-born came to Barns. She is one of the products of orphanage upbringing (about which I am glad to see there are at last some stirrings of the public conscience, if we may judge by the recent spate of letters in *The Times*) and a solemn warning to people who—like myself—are concerned with the bringing up of children in institutions.

But Hugh McGregor's mother was not the product of an orphanage. She enjoyed the privilege of being brought up in her own home, with her own father and mother. Her father was a drunken savage, her mother " no better than she should be," and the " home " was the scene of constant and violent quarelling between them, in which sometimes the neighbours had to separate the contestants. To escape from that home was her only aim—and she finds that in her hurry to escape it she has merely reproduced it. For how many generations, one wonders, does this story go back ? And for how many generations will it continue ? *That* we can do something about. I have suggested how.

These two instances (of many) give the background only of mothers. That is just the accident of war and domestic circumstances which make mothers more available to our enquiries than fathers. In the few cases where we have caught a glimpse of the father's antecedents, much the same sort of thing has been seen.

However angry these parents may make us (and I have not concealed the fact that they make me very angry indeed) it is futile to blame or to condemn them. They need the same kind of sympathetic understanding and help as we try to give their children at Barns. We at Barns, cannot do much about that, but I believe that every such place as Barns should maintain the full-time services of a fully-trained Psychiatric Social Worker for this very purpose —among others. She will not be able to cure the parents of all their troubles—but she will be able to help a good deal, and perhaps act as a buffer between the generations. The parents will be suspicious and will shut up like a clam before anyone who uses even a faintly moral approach. But to anyone who begins to show the slightest understanding of their difficulties and their distress, they will pour out their troubles in a never-ending stream. I myself am the least approachable of men and, as a young man, was much less so. Yet as a " mental health " student I had middle-aged parents pouring out their troubles upon me to the point of embarassment. When that happens a trained and sympathetic worker can very often do a great deal to re-adjust the tangled emotional situations and even sometimes to mend the breaches. Where this proves to be impossible she (it usually seems to be " she." I know of no reason why it should not be " he ") can often facilitate the separation which has hitherto been dreamed of but never accomplished, and which alone can bring peace.

Reggie Mitchell's family illustrates several points that I have tried here to make, and leads naturally on to my next. We never knew his mother, who had deposited him, in his perambulator, on *her* mother's doorstep (subsequently reclaiming and pawning the pram !). I believe she was not at that time married to Reggie's father and whether she has married him since I am not quite clear, but they have lived more or less together ever since, except when they have been in gaol—which has been pretty often. What is the background that has produced this wayward mother? It was, in the first place, a " mixed " marriage, and religion was brought into all the lurid quarrels which provided almost all the emotional warmth the children ever knew. Grannie Mitchell has been married for over 40 years to a man who drinks to excess, is surly and quarrelsome when sober and violent when drunk ; and who at all times is more than a little touched with something very much like religious mania. We know only her side of the story—we do not know what provocations he may have suffered. But for most of her married life she was in misery or in terror. She stayed with her husband at first because of the children, and later because she did not dare and did not know how, to set about getting a separation. We may pause for a moment to wonder what kind of unhappy childhood produced that result in the Grandfather, before passing to look at the result in the Grandson. Grannie tried at first to look after the baby that was abandoned to her but her husband was so violent about what he called " That Protestant bastard " that she had him sent to an orphanage. The Orphanage was a religious foundation and when Grannie took Reg. away at the age of 11, because of the ill-treatment he received there, he was a sour, unhappy bad-tempered and resentful hater of God and man. Grannie found life impossible with such a husband and such a grandson, and the boy came to Barns. I think we were able to help him, though naturally we could not in two years eradicate the result of nine years cruel mishandling.

When the time came for Reggie to leave we were faced with the problem of where he was to live. We had by this time a part-time Social Worker in Hilda Ludlam (Mrs. Gilbert Ludlam) who was in touch with Grannie. She was shocked by the state of affairs she found in the " home" The old couple had not exchanged a word—except sometime in anger—for 10 years. Necessary domestic communication was carried on by means of notes left on the mantelpiece. The old lady was quite fond of Reggie and would have like to make a home for him, but that was impossible. The time for reconciliation was long since passed, but with Hilda Ludlam's help, arrangements were soon in hand for a judicial separation so that the old lady could at least spend her declining years in peace and provide a home for Reg. This story has not, alas, a happy ending. Just when arrangements were in train for the separation, the old man was taken seriously ill, and she naturally could not leave him then.

But we still had to find a home for Reginald—and here, perhaps, I may tell of the Barns Flat.

The Barns Flat is not an official part of our work inasmuch as it was not formally sponsored by the Committee; it is, as it were, a private enterprise on the part of our Chairman, though without the usual rewards of what is commonly conceived by that name. Reggie was not the only boy who had no home to which to return. A flat was therefore secured, just opposite the home of Hilda Ludlam. Certain rooms were sub-let to ordinary tenants, a house-keeper was installed, and the rest of the flat given over to the " Barns waifs." The flat has been the source of endless trouble and worry to all concerned with it ; but it has been the means of salvation already to two Barns boys.

The Social Worker does an indispensable part of our work. She maintains liaison between Barns and the family ; she provides the family history that is so essential if we are properly to understand a boy's history (though lately this has been coming to us through the referring agency—the new Child Guidance Clinic)'; she can often help in the family's domestic difficulties ; she finds suitable jobs for the boys when they leave, and helps them to rehabilitate themselves in the ordinary life of society.

Fourteen is about as unsuitable an age as one could find for effecting a revolution in a person's habits and environment. At this age a boy has entered the stormy and unsettling period of adolescence, but has not yet had time to make any kind of adjustment there. Much of our work would be undone if the boys were not eased gently into their new world. That is the function of the Social Worker.

CHAPTER FOURTEEN

LAST WORDS

> " More devices I tell thee not at this time ; for if thou have grace to feel the proof of these, I trow that thou shall know better how to teach me than I thee. For although it be thus as I have said, yet truly I think that I am full far therefrom."
>
> ANON—" The Cloud of Unknowing."

I MUST make an effort at this point to repress even more than hitherto what little modesty I still retain in order to reply to a criticism that is sometimes made.

Three or four years ago I wrote a book called " The Hawkspur Experiment," in which I recounted something of the work upon which I had been engaged with Q Camps. This book was very kindly received (though alas, its *borrowers* seem to have far outnumbered its *buyers* !) and among several flattering things that were said was one that appeared several times and which, indeed, I had heard before the book was published. The gist of this criticism was as follows. This work about which Wills has been talking, they said, is excellent work. They had every possible sympathy with it, the methods were right and deserved a wider application. But where, they asked, are we to find another Wills ?—the suggestion being, that so far as our work had been successful it was due to my own personal merits and, it was suggested, I was a somewhat exceptional person. It is not enough to dismiss this by saying " rubbish " ; that might cause my kind critics to say, as others did of the anonymous author from whose writings I quoted above— " O Wills *sanctissima, magna est humilitas tua !* "* but it would be no real answer to the criticism, and I think I must try to answer in advance the similar criticism that might be made of this work. My feelings on reading such an opinion are a mixture of gratification at the flattery and irritation at the misconception. Quite apart from the back-hander at my colleagues—both staff and committee— it is really very wide of the mark. I am prepared to concede the possession, perhaps in outstanding degree, of one quality or qualification which may have contributed in large measure to the success of our work, but it is one that anyone may have—I will return to it later. · If our work at Barns has had any success (and I

* *They* said " O Hilton," but they might just as well have said, " O Wills," because neither of us wrote " The Cloud."

am sure it has) it is in spite and not because of my personal qualities. I have most of the commonly recognised disqualifications for dealing with young people or, for that matter, with any people. I am reserved in manner and not easily approachable, and I find it very difficult to make contact with other people, especially with children ; I find that in talking to them I am inclined to be either fatuously facetious or ponderously pompous—I can hardly ever talk to them casually and naturally. I am quick-tempered and my gorge rises far too easily for the preservation of that equanimity that is so essential. Above all (or should I say below all ?) I have that worst possible of vices—I am addicted to sarcasm. I try my best to over-come this weakness and indeed, I believe I do make some progress. But it is so far ingrained in my nature that it sometimes finds expression without my knowledge. When I was doing Settlement work in the East End of London as a young man, I was once—more than once—pursued through several of the streets of Bow by a band of little boys shouting after me, " Sarcy ! Sarcy ! ! " A most humiliating experience—but it did not cure me. I have my good points, too, of course—this is not a masochistic orgy. But if you add to this formidable list of failings all the virtues you can think of—have you then the picture of a man ideally suited for working with difficult children ? You certainly have not. Fortunately several of my colleagues have supplied the qualities I lack, and there is no doubt in my mind that if they had been under the leadership of a man better qualified for working with children, their efforts would have met with even greater success. Provided—and the proviso is of fundamental importance—provided he had also that one virtue to which I have confessed. There is no reason why he shouldn't, but the fact remains that it is not a very common quality, and one of the objects of this book is to increase its incidence. What I confess to, then, is an invincible faith in the methods we have employed and, what is more important, in the spirit which informs those methods. It is a faith that cannot be dimmed by set-backs and apparent failures, because it is based on a firmer foundation than the merely empirical ; and because I *know* that any failures are failures in me, and not in the method.

People often say to me, " I have tried to use your* methods but . . . " That is where we differ. I know no buts. This is a gift which, if you ask, it shall be given unto you, and I hope now that that misconception has been completely cleared.

It may be asked " What then *are* the qualifications to be looked

* I merely quote. They are not " my " methods, of course.

for in the Head of such a place as Barns ? " The personal qualifications are obvious, and some of them I have already, as it were, contra-indicated in speaking of myself. But as to the qualifications that may be gained by education and training, my first desideratum is a negative one. Let him not be a teacher. This will surprise some people—especially after the praise I have bestowed upon some of my own teaching colleagues. But it is not intended as a reflection upon the teaching profession. Indeed I am tempted to say that a bad teacher might make a good warden, but a good teacher—hardly ever. In spite of the greatly widened conception that teachers have, in these days, of their function (and I confess that I sometimes wonder whether there is not a tendency, perhaps, to encroach too far on the sphere of the parent) it remains true that a teacher tends —by training and by the habit of experience—to regard a child as primarily someone to be taught. It is right and natural and very proper that he should do so—just as it is right and proper for the parson to consider us all as so many souls to be saved, and the grocer to regard us as so many customers to be got. He will thus tend— however perfect a man he may be—to confound the good scholar with the good boy, just as the grocer has a predilection in favour of the good customer. However much he may talk of the wide aims of education, his first and most important job is to produce what we might perhaps describe as a " taught " child. The better he is as a teacher, the more keen he is on his job, the more he will subordinate other ends to that. That is what he is trained for and that, if he has a sense of vocation, is his aim in life. He is a specialist. Very good then—let him stick to his last.

I know that in saying this I am attacking a vested interest and a tradition. Most of the Heads of Approved Schools are teachers, and most people will regard this as a perfectly natural thing. " What ! " they will say, " the Head of a school, and not a teacher ? Absurd ! " My point, however, is that it ought never to be a " school " at all. It is all very well to have a teacher in charge of a boarding school (though some of the most famous of them are in the charge of men who are clerics first and pedagogues second), consisting of children with a good home background, who will return to their homes for four or five months out of the 12. That is a school with a kind of inferior, temporary substitute " home " attached, and it is perfectly proper that the Head should be a teacher. But Barns is just the opposite—it is a home with a school attached and that, in my view, is what an Approved School should be. Or, if you like, a number of homes with a school between them. The first function of the Head of such an institution is to provide a home. We have seen (in chapter three) what are the constituents of a good home, and I know of nothing in the training of a teacher that qualifies him to provide these constituents. It is true indeed—alas—that there is at present no academic training that does, but I live in the hope that this evil state of affairs may soon be remedied, and we may have recognised training schools for people who intend to work among the wards of society. In the case, however, of the particular type of child with whom we are now concerned, while it is true that the surrogate father is concerned with every aspect of the boy's life, there are some that must concern him perhaps more than others—I mean those aspects of the boy's character which caused him to become a member of this artificial family. Your warden, too, must be a specialist, and in carrying out his specialist work he will find that he is touching all sides of the boy's life. In this work he may have to call in the help of the teaching staff—but he may equally have to call in the aid of the domestic staff. He should, therefore, be a man of wide interests and experience, with a working knowledge of all that touches the life of the boys in his care, including education in its narrow sense. No academic training, of course, can give him that kind of grasp of the situation, though practical training might. But the one kind of training that is now available, and which (it seems to me) is an indispensable part of your warden's equipment, is what is called Mental Health Training. Your warden should be a trained Psychiatric Social Worker. I hope that when the war is over many more men will take this training than have done so in the past.

I have said that the warden might equally have to call in the aid of the domestic or the teaching staff—but I think there should be very little distinction between them. Certainly your head-teacher will have to specialise in teaching (though not to the exclusion of everything else), your house-matron on her housework and your cook on her cooking. But in my ideal institution there will be a number of young people seeking the kind of widely varied experience I have referred to—trainees—who will participate in a subordinate capacity, in all sides of the work of the house. Thus one of them might be helping in the scullery in the morning and teaching in the afternoon ; another might be helping the warden with his records in the afternoon and supervising some games in the evening . . . We have not been able to achieve that ideal at Barns, but we have achieved the kind of spirit which such an arrangement would ensure. Bill Bell asked one of our domestic helpers to render first-aid to some minor injury he had suffered. She, to tease him, said, " Oh, I couldn't do that. I'm just the scivvy round here. You'll have to find someone more important." "No, you're not," said Billy, "You can do it." "Oh, yes I am," she went on, "I'm just the scivvy. What else am I, then? I'm just the scivvy." "No," said Billy, "We don't have scivvies at Barns. This is not an ordinary place. Barns is different!"

I have one final remark to make, and it is in the nature of an apology. I said on the title page (quoting from John Buchan's first novel, about an earlier inmate of Barns) that my course by the grace of God had had something of a method, which makes the telling the more easy. And so it does. But it also sets many snares for the feet of the unwary. In describing that method, there is a tendency to assume that it has always been applied; one tends to talk about the ideal as if it were the real, and to give counsels of perfection as if we ourselves had unfailingly kept them. I should hate to give that impression—or even to give the impression to our many friends that I was trying to give that impression. I am conscious of having said far too little of our many failures and "warpings past the aim." I have described the will and left my reader to assume a deed that—too often—was not done. "What I aspired to be and was not, comforts me," but I must ask my reader to believe that it has not made me so comfortable that I really imagine our work to have been so near to our aspirations as this account of it may perhaps suggest.

INDEX OF CASES

(The names are of course all fictitious)

GENERAL INDEX

For Product Safety Concerns and Information please contact our EU representative GPSR@taylorandfrancis.com Taylor & Francis Verlag GmbH, Kaufingerstraße 24, 80331 München, Germany

T - #0055 - 160425 - C0 - 216/138/9 [11] - CB - 9781032410463 - Gloss Lamination